Food Allergy Roundtable

A. Anderson

PAPOOSE PUBLISHING LLC

THE BOOK THAT CAN MAKE YOU FEEL BETTER ABOUT
FOOD ALLERGIES

Food Allergy Roundtable is a support-group-in-a-book. Just like a support group, a short story is exchanged. This story allows you to think about your own situation to decide if there is some action you can take to help yourself and your family. It is the perfect guide for a parent or person without the time to attend a support group or read more than a few pages at once.

FOOD ALLERGY ROUNDTABLE

MY PERSONAL SUPPORT GUIDE

A. ANDERSON

PAPOOSE PUBLISHING

ISBN 978-0-692-31087-8

This book is intended to present the research and ideas of its author. If a reader requires personal
advice, he or she should consult a competent professional. The author and publisher disclaim liability
for any adverse effects resulting directly or indirectly from information contained in this book.

Library of Congress Cataloging-in-Publication Data

Anderson, A.
Food Allergy Roundtable.
Includes bibliographical references.
ISBN 978-0-692-31087-8

PAPOOSE
PUBLISHING
www.papoosepublishing.com
Papoose Publishing supports copyright.
Copyright fuels creativity, free speech and new ideas.

Contents

Introduction

The Round Table is King Arthur's famed table in the Arthurian legend, around which he and his Knights congregate. As its name suggests, it has no head, implying that everyone who sits there has equal status.[1]

The term "roundtable" is commonly used to portray a group sitting down to discuss a set of issues, share opinions and ideas. Honest, open, authentic communication is essential. *Food Allergy Roundtable* provides the framework for such a discussion or personal introspection.

A short essay sets the stage—the issue is described. Then through a set of five questions we can each arrive at our own unique best answer to allergy related problems. The busy parent can quickly read a short essay, consider the questions and think about what works best for them. Additionally, the food allergy support group leader can use this book as a tool to facilitate weekly discussions.

Readers will arrive at unique answers for each topic. If all factors, but one, are the same then the answer may be different. For example, two children may have the same allergies, be the same age but one family's relatives may be supportive while the others are not. Therefore the answers to a set of problems might be quite different based upon this diverging factor.

By thinking through situations, considering possible outcomes we can make better decisions and be more prepared to effectively deal with problems that arise in everyday life. This will make us more effective, more relaxed and happier.

Emotional Topics

Feeling Badly

Are you suffering from food allergies? Is your child suffering from food allergies—physically and/or emotionally?

Not being able to eat what everyone else is eating can be emotionally difficult. It can make a person feel different, left out, sad, frustrated and even angry. *"Why me*?" comes to mind. The emotional aspects of having a food allergy are real.

I love my ten year old son's attitude. Somehow, after ten years of having a severe dairy and egg allergy, he's developed a few interesting emotional strengths. Firstly, he often says he likes his dairy allergy and never wants to eat dairy. Secondly, he likes his thin, lean body without the extra pounds that dairy can often pack on. Thirdly, he's tough. He's not a whiner by any means. He gets sick, perhaps more than most. He has seasonal allergies in the spring, where at times his eyes were swollen and red beyond belief. I remember looking at him on the sofa after a particularly bad morning—*"I'm fine*," he said. He wasn't. He had the absolute worst eye allergy attack and cough. We came home to wash his eyes, have him bathe, put ice on and drops in his eyes and let him rest on the sofa. My mother and I just looked at the poor kid. Yes, he is tough emotionally *and* physically.

A couple of weeks ago, we were in church when I perked up by hearing the minister say something about, *"Suffering produces perseverance..."* Yes it does, I thought. My son has suffered—being left out of food at parties and dealing with an overactive immune system. He has been impacted emotionally and physically—an acutely sensitive person in both body and mind. He is amazingly more aware of how others feel than many adults and most children. He asks questions like, *"Mom, when you were growing up, was there something you wanted but never got?"* Wow—no one has ever asked me that! I racked my brain in my response, *"Well yes, I wanted a dog, an open-hole sterling silver flute and to be understood more."*

The point is that suffering, from food allergies, can make you and your child a bit different—*for the better*. More compassionate towards yourself and others, stronger emotionally, accepting rather than angry, and maybe even a bit more grown up than the rest. One of my favorite lines, from *Flourishing with Food Allergies*, is from Dr. Alder where he talks about the greater success in life that these kids will have based upon the suffering and strength they develop from their situation. How encouraging! He saw and recognized that as a pediatrician in his patients. Something good comes out of all of this? Yes!

Parents can support their kids who have food allergies. One simple way to support them is to not eat the foods they cannot eat. I haven't eaten dairy for almost ten years. I've given up eggs too—only ate them once about three years ago, and quite frankly, felt lousy physically afterward—tired, logy. Another way parents can support their kids is to smile and say, *"It's not so bad—who needs dairy [soy, egg, peanuts, tree nuts, fish, shellfish, wheat] anyway?"* Suffering with food allergies can produce strength—enough to smile, accept it and be strong but flexible enough to handle social situations, parties, other people's ignorance and your own attitude with grace. Set a good example for your child and they will learn how to accept and deal with many difficult situations throughout their lives—completely unrelated to allergies.

Roundtable Questions

1. Do you or your child feel badly about being left out of food related events?

2. How do you handle feeling badly?

3. What have you learned about feeling different by having food allergies?

4. Have you developed strengths which influence other areas of your life?

5. Was there something you wanted as a kid, but never got?

Doubting

Just last weekend we went to an end-of-season celebration for our sons' baseball teams. It was held at a small amusement park and there was a short awards ceremony before the BBQ where the kids got medals and small trophies. The boys were thrilled and had a great time. But when the line started for the BBQ, so did my worries.

Our older son remains allergic to dairy and egg now at age seven. I could see the line cooks slapping cheese on every hamburger in sight. Who knew what was in the hot dogs? So I ventured up to the front of the line to see what I could do. I asked if I might be able to see the package for the hot dogs as we've found that milk is an ingredient in many brands of hot dogs. The young girl said she didn't know where the package was and then she turned to ask the guy-in-charge who shouted back to me, "*Hey lady, they're just regular hot dogs!*" Ugh. I gave up and went back to stand with my family in line.

Earlier, at home, I had tried to think this whole thing through and packed a few dairy-free organic hot dogs. They'd been on ice in my backpack for about five hours now—not something I felt good about. So I tried again and went up to the front of the line and asked a kind, older gentlemen if he could warm these up on the grill for me and keep them in the tin foil. He obliged me and about ten minutes later I picked up the hot dogs. But they were not even cooked. They were just the other side of cold, kind-of-almost-warm. My son took a bite or two, but we decided to just make him a hamburger when we would be home. So for now, we gave him a pile of pickles which contented him for the moment.

This was probably one of the more difficult situations that I've encountered with the dairy allergy—one where everyone is eating the same thing and my son cannot participate. At smaller, family BBQs, it is easier to check a label or ask for special consideration. Even storing a hot dog or hamburger from home in a refrigerator is a convenience that can make all the difference—then popping it in a microwave for one minute or so. But these options weren't available to us at this amusement park BBQ.

At times I like these I realize that people just have no idea. It is weird—I too have trouble believing that a common food can be so harmful to some people, like my beautiful son. I know many people, especially those who don't have children with food allergies, have strong feelings of disbelief about others' food allergies. I've even seen stories on TV and on the Internet saying that many, if not most, food allergy tests produce false positives. While there is clearly a lot of doubt, ignorance and skepticism about food allergies, I must admit that I still, at times, struggle with the disbelief grief stage that my husband discusses in his chapter in *Flourishing with Food Allergies* book.

My own disbelief got the better of me this past spring. After my sons had eaten egg baked in bread a few times over the years, I convinced myself they were outgrowing their egg allergy. So I let them try a small bit of hard-boiled egg white not long after Easter. My younger son spit it out saying it was disgusting. My older son said he liked it. Within ten minutes he wanted to vomit and started sneezing uncontrollably. Then within twenty minutes his eyes got itchy, he developed a lot of mucus, became extremely tired and then said his chest hurt. After giving him two doses of antihistamine and talking with our allergist over the phone, I was instructed to give him the Epi-Pen and go to the ER. I am somewhere between ashamed of my actions and dumbfounded by my own disbelief. But the lesson taught us that disbelief is real and dangerous. It also helps me to understand why others feel this way.

Over the next ten, twenty plus years, more and more people will probably develop food allergies. That cook who shouted at me, *"Hey lady, they're just regular hot dogs!"* maybe one day have a child with a food allergy and then maybe he'll think back to all the times he brushed off questions about food that to him may have seemed silly or bizarre. Or news reporters, anchors, talk show hosts who report on food allergy disbelief stories with an air of superiority and insinuation that those who think they have allergies are just a little crazy, may one day understand, when their own children, grandchildren, nieces, nephews or even themselves develop a serious allergy. Maybe when more scientists or government officials' family members develop food allergies then more funding, research and answers will be created. Until then, our virtual food allergy community around the world needs to continue to support one another.

Roundtable Questions

1. Do you sometimes doubt the fact that you or your child has a serious allergy?

2. Do your friends or family members seem doubtful of the allergy(s) and does this make you angry?

3. Have you been able to successfully explain the allergy to someone skeptical?

4. Have you taken a risk by eating an allergen-food because of your doubt?

5. What is the best way to deal with a person who doesn't believe that you or your child has a food allergy?

Staying Calm

Last weekend in an attempt to replace a broken screen door leading out to the deck of our home, I purchased one from a building supply store. It was too short. So in the late afternoon, I drove back to the store to return it. It was hot—very hot. It took about thirty minutes to get there. The air conditioning in the car was broken. It felt even hotter carrying the screen door back into the store. I was hungry, tired, frustrated and disappointed—I actually felt sick to my stomach and a little light headed. After trying to find another door that would fit, I gave up, in despair and felt depressed—surely an overreaction to a screen door problem, but that is how I felt that afternoon.

When I returned home, about one-and-a-half hours later, I found my younger son sitting on a little blue beach chair on the lawn next to the driveway. He was happy to see me—grinning ear to ear and waving to me as I pulled down the driveway. His feet were sort of wiggling back and forth on the green grass in a relaxed, silly way. I thought to myself, *"Wow, I can't believe I just went through what seemed like a nightmare, while my little son had a totally different experience for the past ninety minutes."* I was indeed quite envious.

When I got out of the car, I asked him if he had been here the whole time. He replied, *"Yes Mommy, I was waiting for you. Do you want to play catch?"* I was further stunned that he had been so patient and was so happy despite the heat and the wait. Although I had a headache by this point, I said okay, and we played a bit of catch in the backyard, until I realized I just couldn't even catch the ball that day because I was so exhausted from my own experience and reaction to screen-door-frustration.

So you might ask, *"What does this experience possibly have to do with food allergies?"* Well—it is a vivid reminder that to a large extent we can create our own experiences. While we all must carry the burden of having to deal with food allergies, we can ask ourselves, *"What is my attitude about food allergies in my life? Am I angry? Tired of them? Frustrated? Mad? Feel unfairly burdened? Do I express my frustration at others who are eating peanut butter or dairy near my child? Am I angry with the school? Angry at doctors? Do I feel frustrated towards my own child because of allergies? Do I get angry with relatives during social gatherings when their attitude is not as I'd like?"* In other words, a parent may feel that the food allergies are unfair, so they may therefore carry around a certain amount of resentment and stress that negatively impacts their life, their child's life and those with whom they come into contact.

Instead, consider my little son's take on life: Sitting on the beach chair on the terribly hot day, waiting for ninety minutes for my return—all with a very good attitude. Can we parents find the pleasure in life with all of the good things that we have, despite the food allergies? Perhaps a child has food allergies, but is that child is otherwise healthy, adorable, bright, fun, silly, loving and smart? While social gatherings can be difficult, are there ways to create get-togethers that are more conducive to dealing with food allergies?

How one feels about food allergies in a child, can be controlled to a large extent. A parent can still be careful, but not stressed-out about it. Make the experience of childhood fun, despite the heat (so-to-speak). You can't change it anyway. All you can do is make it better or worse with your attitude and actions. In fact, there are studies that show stress can actually make allergic reactions worse, up to 200% worse! So try removing stress from your allergy situation by working to change your attitude and feelings. Accept the allergies. Deal with the allergies with care, but try to have fun while you kids are growing up. Be like my little six-year-old son who sat waiting patiently and finding fun on the beach chair, doubtlessly getting up now and then to chase a butterfly or look at an ant, and smiling contentedly at me after waiting with anticipation of some more fun upon my return.

Roundtable Questions

1. What is your attitude about your or your child's food allergies?

2. Do you think your attitude impacts how you behave? When? Where?

3. If you did not have to deal with food allergies, how would you be different?

4. Is there a way you can imagine being that different way even *with* the food allergies?

5. Do you believe that changing your attitude will improve your life by reducing your stress?

Feeling Stress

One of the most stressful allergies to have may well be the peanut allergy. While other foods may be more prevalent (dairy and soy for instance are a main ingredient in many off-the-shelf foods) the likelihood that a manufactured food (cookie, cake, cracker) is processed in a facility where other products that include peanuts manufactured is quite high.

Specifically, the same equipment can be used to create a peanut containing granola bar as some peanut-free cookies. But the question remains, was that equipment properly cleaned between manufacturing the granola bars and the peanut-free cookies? For legal and liability reasons, manufacturers will conclude that the equipment may not have been properly cleaned and rightly so include this allergen warning on the label. A few months ago a friend of mine's daughter ate a cookie from her friend's house. The cookie did not outright contain peanuts, but this little girl had a reaction from the cookie, which was manufactured on equipment shared with peanut-containing products.

Although laws have been put into place for the United States, specifically *The Food Allergen Labeling and Consumer Protection Act of 2004* required that by January 1, 2006 manufacturers identify clearly on their food labels if a food product has any ingredients that contain protein derived from any of the eight major allergy foods and food groups: Dairy, soy, eggs, wheat, peanuts, tree nuts, fish and shellfish. But what about food manufactured outside the United States? For instance another friend of mine called Mexico to learn if peanuts ever touched manufacturing equipment that was used to create candy sold here in the United States. Her findings were less than satisfactory— she received mixed messages and felt no confidence that the response was accurate.

So no one argues that stress parents have from dealing with their child's peanut allergy is easy or manageable, but parents can find a bit of solace in several ways. First, read about other parent's experiences and how they have successfully dealt with the peanut allergy in their own children. Secondly, don't give in when selecting foods for your child—continue to select foods that are not manufactured in a facility where peanuts are used. Research what products have peanuts in them and under what names peanut-ingredients hide. Then take it a step further and email the manufacturers asking them to move their peanut containing products to a separate facility. It may not happen right away, but eventually manufacturers will get the message and may reorganize their facilities in the hope of selling more of their products.

Third, consider the advancement made on the peanut allergy front. Reuters recently reports, "*In one study, teams at Duke University in North Carolina and the University of Arkansas for Medical Sciences gave fifteen children tiny, but increasing, doses of peanut powder and compared them with eight children who got a placebo. At the end of the year-long study, children given the treatment were on average able to tolerate fifteen peanuts before having an allergic reaction. 'We started out literally at about a one-thousandth of a peanut and built that up over time,' Dr. Wesley Burks of Duke, who helped lead the study, said in a telephone interview. 'When you take the daily dose it changes your immune system in a certain way and it raises the threshold of how much food it takes to cause a reaction,' he said.*"[2]

Fourth consider other ways to protect your child. For instance, learn your rights by law using a 504 Plan or an allergy action plan for safety in school. Consider contacting your child's teacher to ask if you can give students a presentation on your child's peanut allergy. Take proactive steps when traveling on planes, trains or to other countries to determine the standards and guidelines that can best serve you and your child.

Roundtable Questions

1. Do you feel stress when trying to find safe foods for yourself or your child?

2. Does your stress come from not understanding the ingredients or not trusting the manufacturer?

3. What can you do to improve the chances that the food you or your child eats is safe?

4. Are you willing to make more food from scratch at home to improve the safety of your food?

5. Can you think of ways to reduce your stress in areas where you have little or no control?

Feeling Guilty

As parents, we face many difficult challenges and I know many parents who feel that they could do more for their child—which creates a lousy feeling of guilt. This guilt can lead to frustration because so many of us are busy trying to balance our lives which is a matrix of responsibilities such as taking care of our children, work, homes, finances, friends, relatives and our own health. With the economy in a seemingly constant state of chaos, the financial burdens and stress can compound each of these factors. Then if you factor in food allergies or related disorders of ADHD, autism or asthma, the fear, anxiety and frustration can often feel overwhelming to even the strongest parent. The impact of these problems on families when the children attend day care, school, social events or extracurricular activities can be immense.

Many of us try to make resolutions. Consider this one if you are dealing with food allergies for your child: Stop feeling guilty! Stop assuming any blame for your child's allergies. If you fed them the peanut butter cracker or the almond when they were 'too young' stop thinking that you made some sort of mistake. There isn't enough conclusive evidence in the world of food allergies to know for sure what the right thing is to do. Specifically, should you avoid peanuts or dairy while you are pregnant to avoid creating food allergies in your child? Or should you eat those foods with the hope that those foods will desensitize your baby to an otherwise possible food allergy?

In addition to not feeling guilty about what has happened in the past, consider an additional resolution of acceptance: Accept the reality of your situation and recognize that it could be worse. Specifically, once you accept the food allergy in your child you can: (1) Learn all the names and ingredients that are made from that food allergen (e.g. casein is made from milk protein or arachis is made from peanut); then (2) Take the next step and clean cupboards of all foods containing any ingredient to which your child is allergic. Toss out garbage foods that contain more than five or ten ingredients including corn syrup. To that point, did you know that most corn syrup contains mercury which is a heavy metal that can lead to various disorders such as ADHD and autism?

According to Institute for Agriculture and Trade Policy in 2009, *"Mercury was found in nearly 50 percent of tested samples of commercial high fructose corn syrup ('HFCS'), according to a new article published today in the scientific journal, Environmental Health. A separate study by the Institute for Agriculture and Trade Policy ('IATP') detected mercury in nearly one-third of 55 popular brand-name food and beverage products where HFCS is the first or second highest labeled ingredient—including products by Quaker, Hershey's, Kraft and Smucker's. HFCS use has skyrocketed in recent decades as the sweetener has replaced sugar in many processed foods. HFCS is found in sweetened beverages, breads, cereals, breakfast bars, lunch meats, yogurts, soups and condiments. On average, Americans consume about 12 teaspoons per day of HFCS. Consumption by teenagers and other high consumers can be up to 80 percent above average levels.* [3]

In short, if you are dealing with food allergies, autism, ADHD or asthma stop feeling guilty and start helping your child by clearing out your cupboards of foods that contain the thing he or she is allergic to, as well as high fructose corn syrup.

Roundtable Questions

1. Do you feel like you are to blame for your child's or your own food allergies?

2. How is your guilt impacting how you deal with the food allergies?

3. Do you blame someone else for the food allergies? How is does that impact your relationship?

4. What can you do to stop feeling guilty or placing blame?

5. How will your life and stress level be improved if you accept the allergies as a matter-of-fact and not continue to blame?

Finding Happiness

We were driving in the car coming from baseball practice and going to the pet store for some fish supplies. My younger son, now eight, started talking about his long awaited hamster. I asked him, *"So…you still want a hamster?"* He shouted, *"YES!!"* from the backseat. We have been talking about a hamster for about a year or two now. As an alternative we've built a collection of toy hamsters and tracks during this time—parents' procrastination prerogative. So I replied, *"Well, we did promise you a hamster when you become nine years old—mature enough to clean the cage."* He gleefully yelled, *"My life will be complete!"*

At the ripe old of eight, his life is almost already complete, less a hamster. How great is that? As I relentlessly seek to continue writing and working and finding more studies that interest me, why can't I determine that my life, so full of love and happiness, is complete? It makes me wonder about my attitude towards our food allergies as well—for the past ten years I think I've made every birthday-blow-out-the-candle-wish that the food allergies would—well—just disappear. They haven't. Does that make my life incomplete? Does it make me *un*happy?

No. It better not. There are a lot of things that can go wrong with peoples' lives in this world…from physical, to mental health issues…from accidents to tragedies. Watching television tells us more than we ever want to know about psychopaths, war, poverty, cruelty and all sorts of medical issues that plague us to the point where everyone is impacted by way of our shared and ever-increasing health insurance premiums.

I no longer feel unhappy about our food allergies. I don't even like dairy any more. My older son swears he'll never eat it, even if he outgrows it. He even says he likes his allergies. How can that be? I accept them but only because they've made us healthier—I cook dinner every night. Yes every night, except for when we have leftovers—no take-out, no fast food, no school lunches. I do not always feel like making dinner, but I like eating it. In fact, I love eating it. I don't even like eating out anymore, aside from the social factor, as I prefer my own home cooked mostly organic food. I sleep better, feel better and happier.

So make your life more complete: Don't feel unhappy about food allergies. Make the best of them, cook for yourself and buy the foods you love for your children and yourself. Be safe and don't worry (too much).

Roundtable Questions

1. Do you feel like your life is incomplete?

2. What would make your life more complete?

3. Can you be happy and satisfied in life even with food allergies?

4. Does your attitude affect others around you? If so, how?

5. Would you be able to do something else if you felt happier, even with food allergies?

Staying Hopeful

I received the following story from a mother of an adult daughter who is now grown, healthy and happy. The daughter had severe allergies as a child and was alone in her struggle. Despite the lack of support and being the only child with allergies in their community, this mother successfully raised a daughter who is now twenty-three years old and who has outgrown all of her allergies.

I am posting this story because it provides us with an immense amount of hope. This story shows not only how kids get stronger and can recover from food allergies, but also that we parents today have a lot more support than this mother did twenty years ago. She did it, and we can too. It is important for us to maintain a sense of hope and confidence that our kids will be alright and to give that sense of hope and confidence to our children. Here's her story—

"Twenty-three years ago, my daughter was born full term, but weighed only five and one-half pounds. My pregnancy was miserable, then in her childhood she was allergic to so many things including latex, trees, ragweed, grass, wheat, milk, eggs, cocoa, and more. She was even allergic to the plastic in the bottles so I breastfed her to avoid having her break out in hives all over her face. Similarly, she was allergic to the material in the disposable diapers so I used cloth diapers.

For ten years, I took her to the doctor's four times a week for allergy shots to desensitize her to her allergies—both environmental and food allergens. For years, I watched everything she ate. There were no Epi-Pens back then, so I had bottles of medication that I kept in the refrigerator. If she had a reaction, I had to determine what she was reacting to, mix the appropriate medications and inject it into her myself. The whole experience of her allergies petrified me so that I didn't want to have any more children.

School was very difficult because we knew of no other child who had food allergies. To deal with it, she only ate food from home, never school lunches. But I found the teachers were completely unaware and basically clueless about food allergies. One time, I went into the classroom and found a piece of chocolate cake on her desk for her to eat. I was so angry I threw it. Then I had my daughter moved to a special education classroom so that her diet could be monitored properly by a teacher assigned only to her. No one understood the seriousness of my daughter's allergies—there were children who were lactose intolerant but milk just make them feel sick, it wasn't life-threatening.

I am not sure why she had so many allergies, but I have my theories. Specifically, her father is a Vietnam veteran and was sprayed with Agent Orange. He developed skin cancer when she was a baby. My daughter showed signs of being a late developer and was a little slow in school. But with a lot of help, she graduated from high school early—in the middle of her junior year.

Now she has no allergies! She is only a bit sensitive to the sun and had some fertility problems. She is married and lives on a farm in the Smokey Mountains with her husband and her adopted eighteen-month old daughter. Best part is that she can eat whatever she wants!

Roundtable Questions

1. When you learn of someone getting over allergies do you feel hopeful or depressed?

2. Can you image your or your child's life with no food allergies?

3. What would you do differently if you had no food allergies with which to deal?

4. Do you find yourself avoiding being hopeful so that you or your child are not disappointed?

5. Can you focus on success in other ways despite having food allergies?

Everyday Topics

Increasing Allergies

Recently a friend of mine and I were helping as PTO members with photograph day at our local school. Our responsibilities were to get the kids lined up, organized for their pose and comb their hair—if they wanted us to. I noticed one cute boy whose hair needed to be combed. I asked his teacher if I should comb it and she gave me a quick smile and a resounding, *"No."* Then once he was on the photographer's chair, the photographer went to comb it and the teacher said, *"You can't comb his hair—just take the photo."* She said it with a certainness that was not to be disputed. The photographer backed off and started to take the photo, but the boy began to shake his head back and forth and wouldn't sit for even one second. I'm guessing he is autistic.

During our session, my friend walked over to me from her line of kids and she commented, *"I can't believe the number of kids who are dealing with issues! What is going on?"* She was referring to the kids that probably have ADHD, ADD or autism and who didn't want to be touched, didn't want to smile or needed one-on-one care by a special teacher. I agreed with her, but since I had volunteered previously I wasn't quite as surprised as she was this photograph day.

Why is it, then, that there appear to be so many more kids with issues requiring special care and/or medication than there were twenty or more years ago, when we were kids? What has changed? Based upon my research and reading as a parent and writer, I can list the following things that have changed significantly over the past twenty or so years that can all contribute and impact a child's body and immune system:

- The number of vaccinations has grown a lot:

  - 100 years ago, children received 1 vaccine;
  - 40 years ago, children received 5 to 8 vaccines by age two; and
  - Today children receive 52 vaccines, in the form of 15 shots, by age six months.[4]

- Livestock are given hormones to grow more. Livestock are given antibiotics to treat infections caused by overgrowth.

- Antibiotics were invented 60 years ago. In the last 30 years the use of penicillin-type drugs in farm animals has increased by 600%, and of tetracyclines by 1,500%. The main use of antibiotics in farming is in pigs and chickens.[5]

- Pesticides are sprayed in great quantities on livestock's food and our foods.

- New proteins/DNA structures have been created called Genetically Modified Organisms ('GMOs').

- Heavy metals (antimony, arsenic, bismuth, cadmium, cerium, chromium, cobalt, copper, gallium, gold, iron, lead, manganese, mercury, nickel, platinum, silver, tellurium, thallium, tin, uranium, vanadium, and zinc) exist in our air, water, foods and mass produced toys.

I believe that the net effect of all of these relatively new issues can impact a child's small body in different ways. Each child has a different body—with a different genetic make-up. So each child's body probably handles the onslaught of these impacts differently. Specifically, while one child may develop autism from their body creating a chemical that affects their brain, another child may create IgE antibodies that cause anaphylactic food allergies or a delayed (less obvious but equally devastating) IgG antibody that can cause internal organs to swell like the lungs causing asthma.

It's too early for scientists to prove these ideas. We are in the stage where the reaction has been made, but the cause is not yet discovered. Further, with different bodies and different external factors (the bulleted list above) it is extremely complex to prove: One child can react, but so much differently from the next child.

What is a parent left to do? Not give vaccinations? Not give antibiotics? Not breathe the air or eat our foods? Consider these every day solutions:

1. Buy organic, non-GMO meats and foods not treated with pesticides or given hormones and antibiotics.

2. Only agree to antibiotics if your child is really sick—look for a doctor that agrees and will not just hand them over when your child has a stuffy nose or a virus. Then supplement with probiotics after the run of antibiotics to avoid creating leaky

gut syndrome which can lead to food allergies and related disorders of autism and ADHD.

3. Consider separating and spacing out vaccinations by a week so that the child's body can deal with each one individually. On August 27, 2014, a Center for Disease Control scientist admitted a cover up, *"My name is William Thompson. I am a Senior Scientist with the Centers for Disease Control and Prevention where I have worked since 1998. I regret my co-authors and I omitted statistically significant information in our 2004 article published in the journal Pediatrics. The omitted data suggested that African American males who received the MMR vaccine before 36 months were at increased risk for autism. Decisions were made regarding which findings to report after the data was collected, and I believe that the final study protocol was not followed."*[6]

4. Consider detoxifying your child's body from heavy metals. The medical process for doing this is called Chelation Therapy defined as the, *"[A]dministration of chelating agents to remove heavy metals from the body."*[7] While this therapy uses drugs, we can try eating cilantro (an herb that looks like parsley) to remove mercury, lead and aluminum. *"Chelation therapy using chemicals like EDTA has long been used to help remove these heavy metals, but cilantro is the only natural substance...that has demonstrated this ability...All it takes is adding fresh cilantro to your everyday foods or eating a couple teaspoons of cilantro pesto (1 clove of garlic, 1 cup packed fresh cilantro leaves chopped or blended, 2 tablespoons lemon juice, 6 tablespoons olive oil) a day for two or three weeks."*[8]

Be sure to discuss the antibiotic, vaccination and heavy metal treatments with your doctors. If you find your doctor is not receptive to a discussion, seek out a second opinion. It is important that a parent feel he or she is listened to and has a similar strategy or goal for treating one's child. It may seem like a big step to find a new or different doctor, but it can make a big difference in your child's health and your peace of mind.

Roundtable Questions

1. Why do you think there are more food allergies today?

2. Do you think food allergies can be related to vaccinations and antibiotics?

3. Do you find buying organic, pesticide-free, hormone-free food too expensive or is it worth the cost?

4. Do you think heavy metals can impact food allergies, ADD, ADHD and autism?

5. What can you do to reduce your chances of being impacted by the environment?

Introducing Allergens

There is controversy about when to give a baby or young child peanuts or tree nuts. Some doctors recommend introducing these foods at about one year of age. Others suggest waiting until two or more years of age. Tree nuts include almonds, beechnuts, Brazil nuts, cashews, chestnuts, gingko, hazelnuts, hickory nuts, macadamia nuts, pecans, pine nuts, pistachios and walnuts. Peanuts are not a tree nut—they are part of the legume family as are peas.

As a parent of two food-allergic sons, I am grateful that our sons' allergist instructed us not to give them peanuts or tree nuts until *at least* five or six years of age. I think the old adage, *"An ounce of prevention is worth a pound of cure,"* is perfect advice this situation. Our sons are now six and seven years old. Both had a dairy allergy and egg allergy. One year ago our youngest outgrew his dairy allergy. Neither child has developed a peanut or tree nut allergy—probably because we haven't given them any peanuts or tree nuts.

As a parent of allergic children, I remember feeling the angst of wanting to know if either son would be allergic to peanuts or tree nuts. This need-to-know feeling was strong and the ambiguity bothered me. The ambiguity also bothered me when I explained the situation to others. For example, it was difficult to explain to teachers when they asked, *"Is he allergic to peanuts or tree nuts?"* My answer was and still is, *"My sons don't appear to have an allergy to peanuts or tree nuts but we haven't given them any nor do we plan to until they have fully outgrown their other allergies to dairy and egg."* We've kept them in peanut and tree nut-free classrooms, although they are allowed to sit next to others at lunch who may be eating peanuts or tree nuts.

Normally I don't have the chance to explain the details about our avoidance strategy: Our allergist explained and my research has demonstrated to me that a child who develops food allergies can have an immature or problematic digestive system. For instance, if the child has taken a lot of antibiotics during their young life then the bacteria can be destroyed that normally resides in the child's digestive track or intestines. When it isn't replenished through probiotics (like acidophilus or many other strains), the intestine wall can actually become damaged to the point where tiny holes are created in it. This is called 'leaky gut syndrome' and can be very difficult to diagnose (and see). But one negative result is that food particles can leak through the intestine wall without being properly digested. Then the liver must cleanse the blood of these particles and sometimes the immune system creates antibodies to attack them. Once the antibodies are created the allergic reaction is in place.

Because our sons had food allergies (to dairy and egg) we were extremely wary and afraid of introducing peanuts or tree nuts since the likelihood was high that an allergic reaction would be created. So we waited, and waited, and waited.

Only once our younger son outgrew the dairy allergy just after his fifth birthday, did I give him a peanut. When I did, I made sure it wasn't dry roasted, since those are cooked at such a high temperature that some believe changes the protein and contributes to the creation of a peanut allergic response. Another option would have been to give him boiled peanuts, which are more common in China, and where they have a lower allergy rate to peanuts. Dry roasted peanuts are cooked at temperatures around 400 to 500 degrees. Water boils at around 200 degrees—a substantially lower temperature. Because I had a hard time finding either natural, raw or boiled peanuts, even at our local natural foodstore, I purchased a box of 'natural, organic, raw' peanuts over the Internet from a state across the county. When they arrived, I gave him one-half a peanut each day for several days until I was sure he could tolerate them. I still haven't tried tree nuts. As for my older son, we have not given him peanuts or tree nuts, because his dairy and egg allergy remain present.

Our caution in exposing our sons to peanuts and tree nuts even took place in the allergist's office. When the boys were skin prick tested we opted not to have the peanut or tree nut allergen injected into their skin because we didn't want to expose them to the protein via skin— could this possibly trigger an allergy? Some say yes, others say no. But being the parent of the beloved child, why throw caution to the wind and give it a go? No, we prefer the saying, *"Better safe than sorry."* So we had our sons tested for peanut and tree nuts using the ELISA or RAST blood tests when they were about three or four years old. All blood test results came back negative for allergy to peanuts and tree nuts. But we still didn't give them either of these foods.

Our riskiest behavior will involve occasionally purchasing food that was manufactured in a facility that creates peanut or tree nut products. But for the most part we try to avoid that as well. We will wait until there is evidence that each of our sons' digestive systems is healed and immune systems are less likely to attack protein particles before taking the next steps.

As a mother and researcher of food allergies, I personally think that if a child has other food allergies when they are babies, such as an allergy to wheat, soy, egg, fish, dairy or any food, then that child shouldn't be given the dangerous allergy-foods of peanuts, tree nuts or shellfish until they are older (5+) *and* have outgrown all of their other allergies. As for children without allergies, I'd still wait until the child was at least three or four to introduce peanuts or tree nuts.

Roundtable Questions

1. Do you think introducing allergens early is a good idea or a bad idea?

2. How did your child first become exposed to a food to which he or she had a reaction?

3. Do you think waiting until other allergies are outgrown will help or hurt the situation?

4. How do you feel about the lack of decisive advice from doctors?

5. If you could "do it all over again" what would you do?

Expense of Safe Food

In an already depressed economy, one more strike against a family with young children can be the cost of a food allergy—it can impact both cost of goods and cost of time. Buying dairy-free or egg-free cookies can double the price. Making allergen-free cookies at home takes time—which could be instead spent earning money for a working parent. Furthermore, the cost of an Auvi-Q or Epi-Pen or even the co-payment is not low—depending upon the insurance plan the cost can run from $25 to $60 or more per injector.

Consider the eight major food allergens: Dairy, soy, egg, wheat, peanut, tree nuts, fish and shellfish. In most pre-packaged breads, cereals, cookies, cakes and other off-the-shelf foods, I find dairy, soy, wheat (or gluten) and often egg. Our doctor recommended removing gluten from our sons' diets last winter. Since they already had an egg and dairy allergy, I now needed to find bread that had none of these ingredients. It was easy to find gluten-free bread, but almost all of them had egg, and many had egg and dairy. Oddly, my husband found a brand at a store many miles from our home that had none of these ingredients. Of course a small loaf was $7! With two young boys, a loaf is gone in a few days.

Sometimes I try to make the bread or cookies, but I find that the cost really isn't lower because the dairy-free and wheat-free ingredients are expensive—not to mention the time it takes to buy the ingredients, make the item and clean up. For instance a bag of gluten-free flour can run about $10. It seems that our allergen-free alternatives are roughly twice as expensive as the regular option.

Some of the solutions that I find which do work for us are:

- Purchase a lot of foods in the fruit and vegetable isle;
- Purchase raw, unprepared meats and fish;
- Purchase potatoes, rice, quinoa and rice pasta;
- Purchase mostly water for drinking—some juice and soy or rice milk; and
- Purchase special allergen-free items only for butter and dessert alternatives.

What solutions have you discovered?

Roundtable Questions

1. Have you found that allergen-free foods are more expensive?

2. Do you find yourself making more foods from scratch to save money?

3. What other costs have you experienced due to food allergies?

4. How have you found ways to mitigate or reduce the costs?

5. Do you think it is unfair that allergen-foods are often more expensive?

Food Allergy Labels

Have you ever picked up a favorite food and noticed the ingredients label has changed? Does it now include trace amounts of your or your child's allergic food? Perhaps it now states that it is manufactured on the same equipment as a food containing peanuts, tree nuts, dairy, egg, soy or wheat. Even trace amounts of these foods can trigger allergic reactions or illness for those with celiac disease.

In the past, petitions have been filed with the Food and Drug Administration ('FDA') to require food manufacturers to make these label changes more prominent. Consider writing to the FDA if you think changes to food labels should be clearer.

Consider these issues surrounding food labels:

- Insert a common symbol to indicate the number of food allergens on the front of a package;

- Insert an alert symbol to indicate the ingredients or allergen warnings have changed;

- Force companies to spell out the lump summed ingredients, like 'natural flavors';

- Provide a telephone number for questions about ingredients;

- Provide information if manufactured out of the country and the impact on allergen handling; and

- Provide some clarity on 'manufactured in a facility with other allergens'—is this just a way to avoid liability or could the ingredients be mixed via physical means or by air?

Some folks in other countries have made demands to their governments about the quality of food and the labels. Those governments have enforced changes. For instance, the Bovine Growth Hormone ('BGH') has been banned in other countries (Australia, New Zealand, Canada and the European Union which reportedly includes 28 countries). But the United States' FDA continues to insist it is safe, despite evidence that it causes cancerous cells to grow.

Write to your government and ask for changes!

Roundtable Questions

1. Should food manufacturers be forced to indicate changes of ingredients in a prominent way?

2. Should there be additional warnings for other foods instead of just the big 8 (dairy, wheat, egg, fish, shellfish, wheat, soy, peanuts, tree nuts)?

3. Should food manufactures be banned from using lump sum ingredients like spices or natural flavors?

4. Should foods from other countries have a screening process so that they meet requirements of the receiving country's allergen label?

5. Should the United States ban BGH like the 28 countries in the European Union?

Outgrowing Allergies

Is there a chance that children can outgrow their food allergies? It appears so, based upon official studies and unofficial stories. For instance, my younger son, who just turned five, had his annual allergy skin prick test just before his birthday. He had shown positive for egg and dairy since he started skin prick tests when he was two. We never actually fed him these foods, except one bottle of cow's milk formula the nurse gave him (by mistake) on the day he was born.

Now finally, his skin prick test for dairy, at age five, came back negative. We were then referred to a larger office of allergists where they conduct challenge tests. But before the doctor to whom we were referred would do a dairy challenge test, she insisted on a blood test. She said that only if both the skin prick and the blood test come back negative is there a solid chance that the child has fully outgrown the allergy. So two weeks later we had the blood test done and another week passed when we learned that the results were negative, which was good news.

We scheduled our challenge test and my son had to miss a day of school. It lasted three long hours, but my son passed the test and was able to consume six ounces of organic 2% cow's milk in increasing amounts over the first two of the three hours. After the test, I was exhausted—emotionally. I had tried not to get too excited, for fear of disappointment, but when I found out he was okay, the thrill I had dreamed of was lacking for me. I think I had prepared myself for failure, so was somewhat hardened which left the happiness factor out in the cold to a certain extent. It took about a week before I shared the good news with my friends and some others. Yes, this reaction is weird, but that's what happened. Now about a month later, I feel relief, and I guess happiness, but I think I am still quite guarded, probably from a continued fear of disappointment.

Enough about me, upon seeing my older son get off the school bus, I wondered, "*What do I tell my six-and-one-half year old who is still allergic to dairy?*" Well, I told him that he should be happy for his little brother. He responded, *"Oh!"* and his eyes lit up a bit—very sweet. Then I said, *"And because your little brother has outgrown his allergy to cow's milk it could mean that you are next because you and he are so much alike."* It is wrong to set up this hope? Coincidentally, a couple of weeks before all of the success of my younger son, his older brother said for the first time, *"I wish I didn't have food allergies,"* one night just before going to sleep. I assured him he would outgrow them someday. Then sometime over the next week, during dinner, something inspired me to tell my boys that food allergies really aren't that bad because there are a lot worse things that can happen to a person—then I proceeded to list them off. Not sure this was the right thing to do, but it did stop any further whining about our situation.

I can only attribute my younger son's success in outgrowing his allergy to strict avoidance. My husband and I are extremely careful about not giving him any foods that contain dairy, even in trace amounts. Other than that, we try to reduce stress in our lives as much as possible and give our kids their time to be quiet and play as they wish—which supports the toxic load theory, discussed in *Flourishing with Food Allergies*. Sometimes this means not signing them up for another session of soccer or t-ball so they can relax on Saturday mornings rather than rushing out for yet another activity. Also, I faithfully give my son a dairy-free multi vitamin and dairy-free probiotic supplement every morning.

What about other food allergies? What are the average rates for outgrowing those?

- 80% or 'most' of children will outgrow these allergies by the time they are 16 and as early as age 3: Dairy (cow's milk products), egg, soy and wheat;[9], [10]

- As many as 20% of children will outgrow their allergy to peanuts;[11]

- Less than 10% will outgrow their allergy to: Tree nuts (almonds, Brazil nuts, cashews, hazelnuts (filberts), macadamia nuts, pecans, pine nuts (pignolias), pistachio nuts and walnuts. [12] Note: Peanuts are part of the legume family and are not considered a tree nut.)

As for fish and shellfish, most research says the allergy is normally life-long. But perhaps some reactions can be outgrown. For instance, my father had reactions of severe nausea and vomiting after eating scallops and shrimp as a teenager and in his early twenties. He recalls, *"The first instance was in New York. I was about sixteen years old when I went to lunch with one of my friends. Then I went back to work. Once at work I vomited so badly I had to go home. Another time was when was in college when I was about twenty years old. I ate at the college restaurant and vomited again. In both cases the other people had the same food and were fine, so I concluded that the food wasn't bad—it was* my *reaction to it. So I swore scallops and shrimp off."* The good news is that in his mid-twenties, my mother convinced him to try eating these scallops one night. He tried and he was fine! Over the past forty-five years, he has been able to eat scallops and shrimp without a problem.

Roundtable Questions

1. Should a parent instill hope in their child that the child will outgrow a food allergy?

2. Is strict avoidance of an allergen the best course of action to outgrow a food allergy?

3. Is it dangerous to give a child very small doses of an allergen to desensitize them?

4. Should food allergy challenge tests be done only if the blood and skin prick tests are both negative?

5. Is it unfair to siblings to ban foods that others in the family are allergic?

Tree Nut Allergies

Tree nuts include the following nuts that are grown from trees: Almonds, beechnuts, Brazil nuts, cashews, chestnuts, gingko, hazelnuts, hickory nuts, macadamia nuts, pecans, pine nuts, pistachios and walnuts. Peanuts are not a tree nut—they are part of the legume family as peas.

"About 9 percent of children will outgrow tree nut allergies," according to a study led by Robert A. Wood at Johns Hopkins University School of Medicine, *"58% of children with tree nut specific IgE levels of less than 5 kilounits per liter passed an oral challenge. Based on these findings, researchers recommend that children with a current tree nut allergy be reevaluated periodically by their allergist/immunologist to assess whether they have developed a tolerance and whether an oral challenge should be given. While an ideal cut-off has not been established, researchers suggest that oral challenges should be considered in children four years and older, and who have less than five kilounits per liter of tree-nut specific IgE in their blood...[But] children who are allergic to multiple types of tree nuts are unlikely to outgrow their allergy."*[13]

That begs the question, *"What is there to do for the remaining ninety percent of children who do not naturally outgrow a tree nut allergy or have multiple types of tree nut allergies?"* It can be stressful for parents and children who have allergies to these nuts which may be found as ingredient in everything from health food bars, bouillon and Worcestershire sauce to non-food items like hackysacks, beanbags, draft dodgers or bird feed. Aside from avoiding tree nuts, there is more hope for a cure. In 2010 FAAN awarded Dr. Stacie Jones of Arkansas Children's Hospital to receive grant money for the purpose of developing, *"Tree nut-specific immunotherapy for people who have multiple tree nut allergies. Considerable progress has been made using oral immunotherapy approaches for other food allergens, but this will be the first study to focus on the treatment of multiple tree nut allergies."*

Roundtable Questions

1. Do you think that manufacturers should be required to indicate if a food, like nut shells, is used in a non-eatable product?

2. Should the government create an initiative to help people outgrow tree nut allergies?

3. Should manufacturers come together to help people outgrown tree nut allergies so they can increase sales?

4. Should peanuts be included in tree nut categories due to ignorance about their true classification?

5. Should make up or sunscreens be required to ban ingredients from tree nuts, peanuts, dairy or other allergens?

School Topics

Starting Pre-School

If your child is starting pre-school or kindergarten with food allergies, you as a parent will likely be apprehensive. There is comfort in knowing that you are not alone—other parents have successfully dealt with the situation. Furthermore, there are laws that support your concerns.

Here are some suggestions for setting up a safe environment for your new-to-school child:

1. Meet with the school to learn their practices for keeping children with food allergies safe;

2. Ask the school if every teacher and supervisor has training and the authority to administer antihistamine and epinephrine using both the Epi-Pen and Auvi-Q injector types;

3. Ask if there have been any food allergy incidents and how each was handled;

4. Learn if the children will be eating in a supervised and controlled environment or more free-form;

5. Ask if other parents allowed to bring food in for the entire class and whether you will be notified ahead of time to provide your child with a safe version of the food; and

6. Try to get some references of other parents whose food-allergic children have attended the school—call or email them to find out how satisfied they were with the school or what warnings they might have.

Any reputable pre-school or school must ask for signed medical permission forms for the authority to give a child medication. If the school states they do not need these—beware—this is not the norm.

One last item is to purchase a fun, cooled lunch box so that you can pack a great snack and lunch for your child. Kids like options—just like adults. Lots of little choices can be more fun for the children than a sandwich, for instance. Perhaps little containers of crackers, fruit, vegetables, pretzels, cookies and a few protein options (e.g. rolled turkey, sliced sausage) would be more appetizing for your child. Don't forget to ask your child what they would like to eat while at school—they have opinions and may simply not think to volunteer them. I've learned a lot just by asking!

Roundtable Questions

1. Should a school cater to food-allergic children by not allowing certain foods in school or classrooms?

2. Should all personnel be trained on the administration of epinephrine? If they are not, how can that be remedied?

3. Would it be helpful if epinephrine is made available in various locations throughout the school (not just the nurse's office)?

4. Would you trust allergen-free lunch options, if they were offered by the school?

5. How accountable would you make teachers for ensuring safe food-related parties or projects in the classroom?

School Buses

Have you investigated how a school bus emergency would be handled with respect to an allergic reaction?

Is your child allowed to carry epinephrine on the bus? If so, is the bus driver trained and authorized to administer it? If not, do the local ambulances carry epinephrine? What is their average response time? What is the method of communication between the first responder or ambulance and the school personnel? How will the first responder be made aware that your child has food allergies if the child is not able to communicate this effectively?

I asked these questions of the school, bus company and local fire department. The fire chief took it upon herself to work out a plan with the others to handle school bus emergencies especially with respect to health issues such as food allergies and asthma. It took from September through November to arrive at the plan and even a bit longer for all aspects of the plan to be put into place. It is important to be respectful and patient when working with these authorities. It may take several months to work out a plan. Here is a summary of the plan that was worked out in our town.

Summary: Over the past three months an effort was made to review and put into place a process for handling an emergency on a school bus. A special consideration was made to discuss how children with health issues would be identified and treated in such an emergency. These health issues might include food allergies, asthma or diabetes.

Purpose: This emergency plan addresses the issue of if there is a bus accident or other emergency, how would the emergency responders identify which children have special health considerations or needs?

Plan: It was decided to establish a password so that the Officer-in-Charge ('OIC') can provide the password when communicating with the school personnel at the time of an accident. Once the password is communicated, the school personnel will access the database on the computer system at the school. This database contains the health information of students as provided by the parents via the health information forms. If parents do not fill out or submit the forms, then their children's health information will not be in the database. Parents can ask for a form to resubmit or update their children's health information at any time. This database can sort the students according to which bus route they are on. So if a bus has an accident, then all students on that bus (e.g. Bus 9) along with the health information can be pulled up and provided to the OIC at the scene of the accident. (It was decided not to store this information on the bus because bus routes may change at the last minute due to breakdowns or change in personnel.)

The current method of communication will be cell phones. Regular radios will not be used because they are not private and would therefore violate HIPAA laws. Funding is being sought for purchase the private channel over which the radio can be used to communicate the health information. This solution will provide more reliable communications than cell phones and will be in compliance with HIPAA since it will be over the private channel. The cost is about $3,000. This cost has been submitted as a budget item and will need to go through the process of getting placed into the budget. In the meantime, the cell phones will be used so that information can be obtained if needed. A dispatching policy is now in place to notify the proper individuals at all schools when a bus accident is reported.

A first responder is the police, fire department or ambulance. The only medication that the police or fire department can administer is oxygen. Our town's ambulance has EMTs, not fully trained paramedics, but the EMTs are trained on the use of Auvi-Q or Epi-Pen injectors and medication for diabetics and they carry these medications in the ambulance. If this higher level of medical care or medication is required, then the R5 ambulance out of the neighboring city is dispatched, which takes about 12 to 15 minutes on average to arrive at the scene. This ambulance has fully trained paramedics.

Time can be critical if the emergency on the bus involves certain health issues. For instance, if a child has an allergic reaction and is going into anaphylactic shock, they need to receive a shot of epinephrine from an Auvi-Q or Epi-Pen within 20 minutes. Because the number of children with food allergies is rising at a rate of 20% per year, parents are bringing this health issue to the attention of the officials so that an increased awareness can be had. Currently 4%-8%, between 1 in 13 or 1 in 25, of children have severe food allergies— which is about three million nationwide. Other health issues that have critical timeframes are asthma and diabetes.

Open Issues: The above plan was discussed and agreed upon, but two outstanding issues remain open: (1) One is a budgetary item for a private radio channel—in the meantime there is a workaround (cell phones); (2) The other is the reliance upon parents to provide the health information form to their schools so that the school's database system has up-to-date health information on the child. In other words, no matter how good the plan is, if the parents have not provided the information, then the children's health issues will not be known to the emergency responders. For this reason, a health information form will be resubmitted to each of the parents in the region's four schools, along with this summary and the request for the information to be completed and sent back to the school.

Roundtable Questions

1. Should emergency first responders (e.g. police) have access to school health records?

2. Would you recommend that school bus drivers be trained on the administration of various medications such as epinephrine?

3. Is the school responsible for the safety of the children riding the bus?

4. If the bus company is a 'paid-for-hire" service of the school, should the bus company be responsible for safety or the school or both, i.e. who is ultimately responsible?

5. Do you think that tax payers' dollars should cover special medical needs, like having nurses on field trips or special lunches, like those with special education needs are covered?

School Checklist

Starting school or going back to school for a child with food allergies can be a stressful event for parents. While we want our children to be safe, we also don't want a reputation as a crazy mom or dad. Here are some checklist items to make sure you've done all that you can to help get your child off to a safe start. Even if you are a few weeks into the school year, it isn't too late to do any of these items now.

School Checklist:

1. Set up a private meeting with you and your child's teacher. At that meeting, give the teacher a piece of paper that you prepare on the computer or in your own hand writing. List the child's name and if possible attach a photograph to the paper. If doing it on the computer, go to the 'Insert' menu and insert a 'picture from file.' Ask the teacher to put it on the wall so that even a substitute teacher will be able to quickly identify your child. Then list all of the food allergies that affect your child. If they are allergic to tree nuts then list each specific nut individually—there is often a lot of confusion about what tree nuts include and the difference between them and peanuts. Also ask the teacher to notify you of all food-related events prior to them occurring so that you can send in some safe food treats for your child, such as a peanut-free cupcake for a birthday party to be held in the classroom.

2. Ask the school's nurse to provide you with an Allergy Action Plan template that you can fill out. This plan lists the food allergies and medications that the child should be given. Make sure the school nurse has medications that are not expired and that list the amount needed for your child based upon your child's weight. Specify the hospital you'd like your child to go to in case of an emergency. For more detailed instructions, you may opt to prepare a 504 Plan. Look this up on the Internet for some examples. You may need the help of an attorney for a 504 Plan.

3. Ask the school's principal if other personnel at the school are trained in administering Auvi-Q or Epi-Pen injectors. Normally the teachers and the principal should be trained and should know how to find the epinephrine for your child, if the school

nurse is not available for some reason. Make sure you go back and question the teacher as to whether he or she knows where the Auvi-Q or Epi-Pens are stored and how to locate your child's epinephrine in case of an emergency.

4. Ask the manager of the cafeteria what the procedures are for peanut-free/tree nut-free tables. Ask if they accommodate other allergies at tables such as for dairy or egg. Find out if there is an 'emergency' sign or symbol that your child can make/do should they feel like they are having an allergic reaction and need special help. For instance, instead of raising just one hand, perhaps they could put both hands up to indicate to the teacher-on-duty in the cafeteria that they need help fast.

5. Ask your local emergency (fire/ambulance) department if the ambulances they drive carry epinephrine. Let them know that your child is riding the bus and that the bus driver doesn't have an Auvi-Q or Epi-Pen or permission to administer it. Ask them how they communicate with the school to identify medical issues in children, if the child is unable to communicate his or herself.

6. If you are having a problem doing any of these items above because the personnel are not being respectful, responsive or receptive then contact a lawyer for a consult. That lawyer may be able to prepare a short letter to send to them so that they know you are serious and so is the food allergy issue. It may cost you a fee of say $60 for the letter—check with the attorney before you take too much of his or her time, and let them know your budget and concerns.

Don't be shy about contacting school personnel about your child's food allergies. You are protected under the Americans with Disabilities Act ('ADA') which is a civil rights law that gives you the right to ask for changes where policies, practices or conditions exclude or disadvantage you or your child. Plus Section 504 of the Rehabilitation Act of 1973 further provides you with rights for food allergies. Section 504 prohibits discrimination on the basis of disability in employment and education in agencies, programs and services that receive federal money. In both the ADA and Section 504, a person with a disability is described as someone who has a physical or mental impairment that substantially limits one or more major life activities, or is regarded as having such impairments. Breathing, eating, working and going to school are 'major life activities.' Asthma and allergies are still considered disabilities under the ADA, even if symptoms are controlled by medication.

Roundtable Questions

1. Should the school have emergency procedures in place for children with food allergies?

2. Should children be allowed to carry an Auvi-Q or Epi-Pen in school or on the bus? At what age?

3. Do you think it is fair that parents need to contact (and pay for) lawyers for the creation of a 504 plan?

4. Are food allergies a disability? What is a disability?

5. Do schools have the right to push-back and limit the protections if too expensive or cumbersome?

Teacher Communique

Consider giving your child's teacher an allergy notice that contains specific information about your child's allergies as well as his or her photograph. It will make it easier, and safer, when a substitute teacher is supervising your child's class—she (or he) can see the child's face along with the allergies and likely symptoms of a reaction. Here's a sample form:

Child's Name: Teacher's Name: Grade Class

Food Allergies:

- Dairy (milk, cheese, yogurt, etc...see list below)
- Egg
- Tree Nuts
- Peanuts

[INSERT PHOTO HERE]

Reaction Description:

Reaction to ingesting the food only (no reaction to touching or breathing in the food):

- Mucus that causes coughing, sneezing, nausea
- Hives or rash on face or body
- Itchy face, nose or eyes, possible swelling

Classroom Food:

Snacks that do work are: plain potato or corn chips (no flavors like sour cream or even salt and vinegar which sometimes contain milk), plain pretzels, fruits, veggies, fruit pops, fruit rollups.

If there is a party or food event planned, please notify _____ ahead of time so that she can send in food for that is similar to the food that will be served at the party, like cookies or a cupcake for instance. The contact email is _____ and the phone is _____.

THANK YOU!

AVOID ALL DAIRY INGREDIENTS INCLUDING:		AVOID ALL EGG INGREDIENTS INCLUDING:	AVOID ALL TREE NUTS AND PEANUTS
beverage	lactose	albumin	Almonds
whitener	malted milk	egg solids	Beechnuts
butter	margarine	egg white	brazil nuts
butter oil	milk powder	egg white solids	cashews
calcium ca-	milk solids	egg yolk	chestnuts
seinate	non-fat milk	globulin	gingko
calcium lac-	non-fat milk solids	lecithin (maybe)	hazelnuts
tate	potassium caseinate	livetin	hickory nuts
caramel	ready sponge	lysozyme	macadamia nuts
casein	skim milk powder	ovalbumin	pecans
caseinate	sodium caseinate	ovoglobulin	pine nuts
cheese	sour cream	ovomucin	pistachios
cream	sweet whey powder	ovomucoid	walnuts
custard	vegetable fats	ovotransferrin	
curd	whey	ovovitelia	Peanuts are not a
demineralised	whey protein	ovovitellin	tree nut--they are
whey	whey solids	powdered egg	part of the legume
fromage frais	yogurt	silici albuminate	family as are peas.
galactose	*Doesn't include:*	simplesse	
ghee	*calcium citrate*	vitellin	
lactobacillus	*calcium carbonate*	Whole egg	
lactalbumin	*potassium lactate*		
phosphate			
lactalbumin			
lactate			
lactic acid			
lactoglobulin			

Roundtable Questions

1. Should teachers be formally trained on food allergies, not just administering epinephrine?

2. Should schools initiate standard parent meetings for children who have food allergies?

3. Do other parents in the classroom have a duty to avoid the allergen foods for parties?

4. Is the school responsible for training substitute teachers on medical issues of students in the classroom?

5. If substitute teachers are less trained than regular teachers is the school liable if there is a problem?

Nut Free Lunch Tables

Does your school have a peanut and tree nut-free lunch table?

With the numbers of school children with food allergies increasing each year, perhaps it is time to rethink the peanut/tree nut-free lunch table. What if schools set up the opposite table: The peanut/tree nut table? Specifically, if the non-allergic child who is eating a peanut butter sandwich or a granola bar containing tree nuts were to sit at the table designated for peanut and tree nuts it would contain or limit the allergen contaminants to that table, thus allowing the allergic children to sit with their classmates as they choose.

This shift in thinking could help children who have the allergies to these highly allergic foods to feel more integrated rather than segregated. It would allow the children a chance to socialize with children who they normally wouldn't sit near, i.e. not just those classmates who have similar allergies.

Perhaps suggesting this idea to school personnel will get the ball rolling in that direction so eventually this policy could be put in place.

Roundtable Questions

1. Is it fair or just safe that children with peanut or tree nut allergies be forced to sit at a special lunch table?

2. Would having children who eat peanut or tree nut products sit at a special lunch table be safer or fairer?

3. Should schools be allowed to determine the lunch table rules or should the rules be state or federally mandated?

4. Should certain foods be outlawed at schools or on planes, like peanuts, or on a case-by-case basis?

5. With the rise in severity of other allergens, should dairy or egg or soy free lunch tables be set up as well?

School Parties

How do you handle all of the birthday parties and holiday parties that occur in the classroom at your child's school if he or she has food allergies? It seems that with twenty to thirty kids in each class, every month has about two birthday parties with cupcakes or cake. If it isn't a birthday party, there is a party being planned for Halloween, Thanksgiving, Christmas or Hanukah, St. Valentine's Day, St. Patty's Day or even Easter.

If you child has allergies to dairy, egg, soy, wheat, peanuts or tree nuts (almond, beechnuts, Brazil nuts, cashews, chestnuts, gingko, hazelnuts, hickory, macadamia, pecans, pine nuts, pistachios and walnuts) then sharing party treats like cupcakes, cookies or other snacks can be not only difficult but downright dangerous.

I have two boys in school at this time: One is in kindergarten and the other is in first grade. Both boys have had allergies to dairy and egg pretty much since birth and we've avoided giving them any peanuts or tree nuts in a hope to fend off developing an allergy. (We will try those foods when they are older and hopefully outgrow the first two.)

My younger son outgrew his dairy allergy in the beginning of his kindergarten year. His egg allergy appears to be mild enough to allow him to eat cooked eggs in baked goods. So over the past five months, after discussion and letter from his allergist, his teacher and I allowed him to participate in eating the party food prepared by other mothers. His classroom is peanut-free and tree nut-free, so there was little risk of those allergens being included in the baked treats. Thankfully, he has been able to eat the foods and only vomited once after eating a cupcake. I think he had a little stomach bug as well on that day, so afterward, his teacher and I decided it was probably the combination of the richness of the cupcake mixed with an already upset tummy to cause this problem.

But what if your child has full blown allergies? Well my older son remains severely allergic to dairy and egg and we avoid all peanut and tree nuts. Anyone who has baked a cookie or a cake knows that butter and eggs are almost always called for in these treats. I know from first-hand experience that it can be difficult to make a cake rise without eggs and make a cookie stay cohesively together without eggs. What about taste? Butter is yummy and makes everything so tasty.

Here's what has worked for me: Last year, when he was in kindergarten, I made a stash of allergen-free cupcakes, frosted and put them in the freezer. Then when the teacher sent home the list of birthdates, I carefully marked each day on my calendar to remind myself to put a cupcake into his snack bag so that he did not feel left out. Now that he is in first grade, I volunteered to be Room Parent because I have a little more freedom now that my younger son is in school too. Room Parents have the responsibilities of planning the parties.

My Co-Room Parent and I create a party plan a couple of weeks beforehand. I normally take over the communication of food items to the other parents, with special care to those who have food-allergic children. If I am to make the cupcakes for the entire class, I will email the recipe to the parents of food allergic children and assure them that no peanuts or tree nuts come near the countertop. In fact we don't even have them in our house. If a candy item is planned, I will ask the parent to communicate in email the ingredients and any allergen warnings. I often ask the allergy-parents to do the purchasing, since they are more aware of checking the labels. We always cc the teacher on the email so that she knows which children can have what foods.

Even with a lot of planning and care, I learned that sometimes I need to pick up the phone and call the other parents. Last month it was my son's seventh birthday. So I made cupcakes for the class and emailed the recipe to those mothers whose child has food allergies. One mother said, *"Great, my daughter can eat it."* Another mother said, *"No, it contains soy."* But there was <u>no</u> response from a third mother. So the day of the party, the daughter of that third mother came up to me and said, *"Can I have a cupcake?"* I said, *"Well it has no peanut or egg, so it might be okay, but your mommy never wrote back to my email so perhaps you shouldn't have it."* The teacher agreed through a nod of her head. We tried to praise the little girl for being so grown up about asking.

I felt so terrible for that little girl. The other kids loved the cupcakes. One boy said it was the best cupcake he'd ever had in his whole life. After the cupcakes were gone, that little girl came back over to me and said, *"I bet those cupcakes were really good."* Ugh! I felt even worse. While I wanted to be angry with her mother for not getting back to me, I realized that really doesn't help the little girl. So I tried to think about what I could do to prevent this from happening again. I decided that I would call the mother in the future to make sure she got the email and decided one way or the other if her daughter could eat the cupcake.

So now it will be Valentine's Day in a few days and the big party at school is tomorrow. As I promised myself, I followed up with that mother of the little girl carefully and this time she responded. She agreed to allow her daughter to eat the dairy-egg-peanut-tree nut free cupcake I am making and I forwarded that email to the teacher. I feel so much better about the whole thing. I still feel a bit bad for the girl because I know she has dealt with a lot of disappointment and will in the future, because her mother doesn't put a priority on this issue—and she is even a nurse—but at least in my own little way, I am making a tiny little difference in that girl's day tomorrow.

Making cupcakes, cookies and cakes isn't hard. It might take a few practice attempts, but don't despair, once you find *one* recipe that works, that's all you need. There are a lot of great recipe books out there and it is worth ordering one or two. Here are the basic rules I use:

- Never use any nut, peanut or nut extract period;

- For dairy-free items, I use the Earth Balance non-GMO buttery spread. It is all vegan and tastes great. Beware of other margarines—many contain cow's milk product! Look at the ingredients including casein;

- For egg-free items, I will use one of the following substitutes to try to make stuff rise and stick together: 1T of applesauce for each egg (holds stuff together),or¼ banana for each egg (holds stuff together and makes it moist, a little banana taste), or 2.5 tsp. baking powder + 3T oil +3T water mixed together (keeps stuff soft and rises). Beware of 'egg substitutes'—many actually contain egg products, especially in the egg section;

- Always read the ingredients carefully and the allergen warnings. There are detailed lists of ingredients in Chapter 38 of *Flourishing with Food Allergies* that come from the big 8 allergens. For instance casein is a dairy ingredient that must be avoided for those allergic to dairy because it is the protein part of the dairy—the worst part for those with allergies to dairy.

It is extra work, but work well worth the effort. You will become a better cook. You will feel better about your child's situation. Your child will appreciate it.

Roundtable Questions

1. Should parties at schools be banned?

2. If parties are banned, what are the pros and cons for the children? The adults?

3. If parties are not banned, should teachers and room parents cater to the food-allergic children?

4. Should notices about allergies be communicated to all parents?

5. If parents do not comply with classroom food allergy rules, what should the consequences be?

Social Topics

Invisible Disability

Last week I went for a swim. I was about half way through my normal regimen of laps and noticed another person coming into the pool area. The person was a young woman with dark hair in a ponytail who was walking with crutches because she had an amputated leg. I immediately felt a combination of sympathy and awe—wondering if she had been injured in the war and how she is coping. I continued to swim while she jumped into the pool and started to swim in the lane next to me.

As I continued to do my laps, I began to think about how people react when I tell them that our son has severe food allergies to dairy and egg. The emotions range from sympathy to a sort of disbelief. Sometimes the sympathy is over the top—almost a pitying, *"How can you live like that?"* Other times the sympathy is tainted with 'schadenfreude,' that practical German word missing in our English language for the often-present pleasure that some folks take in watching the misfortune of others. Don't believe it? Just watch the evening news—it is almost all bad news.

Sometimes the disbelief can insinuate that a parent or person is over-protective, over-cautious or just a little bit peculiar to be worrying about a harmless food. These folks often forget about the food allergy when they visit with peanut butter candy on their lips or hands and a sense of careless disregard. Then when gently reminded of the dangers, the person might reply, *"Oh yeah, that's right—I totally didn't think of that."*

In contrast to the brave woman who swam next to me in the pool, where there is no getting around her disability, the invisible disability of food allergies is laden with not just the food allergy itself, but the various attitudes that people take towards it. I think that it can be best summed up by the phrase, *"If you can't see it, don't believe it."* The bottom line is that dealing with a food allergy is not just dealing with the allergy itself but the social aspect of it as well—which can be equally if not more troubling at times.

What are the resulting feelings? I must admit I feel much more protective about my older son than my younger son, since my younger has outgrown the allergies. I do not want my older son to sleep over someone's house—I would worry all night long. Upcoming field trips—these frighten me too—especially the overnight ones. I was extremely nervous when my son went to kindergarten, but now that he is in fifth grade, I have confidence in the school's systems and nurse to take care of the children. It is the ad hoc activities that give me pause—like field trips, parties and after school events, where carefully planned controls are thrown by the wayside. That is when people, food, situations arise that can be dangerous—and the invisible disability can't be seen nor easily handled by those that are not trained.

Roundtable Questions

1. Should we refer to food allergies as a disability? What benefits are derived from that?

2. How do you deal with others who don't want to help out with the food allergy situation—parents at school or unsupportive people?

3. Should we change our decisions about what we or our children can or cannot do based upon having a food allergy?

4. If there is a special field trip or dinner that you or your child wants to attend, should special accommodations be made for us or are we responsible?

5. Should we have to file a 504 disability plan to have special considerations for various events?

Trustworthy People

As I drove home from my technical writing job today on the interstate going at around 60 to 65 mph there were a lot of cars in the two lanes that fanned out to three or four then back to two. With both hands on the wheel, I listened to my favorite Mozart CD and drove. I glanced in my rear-view mirror and saw a woman behind me who was talking with a man who wore a dark business suit, white shirt and red tie. She quickly turned to look at him and seemed very interested in carrying on the conversation making some small hand gestures as she spoke. She made me a bit nervous. Minutes later, I saw two young men in a small, older car closing in quickly on me seemingly within feet from my rear bumper—much too close for my comfort. In both cases, I put on my blinker and moved to the next lane to get away from what I perceived as dangerous drivers.

As I continued to drive, it occurred to me that my driving attention includes a significant effort of watching the behavior of other drivers and reducing my risks by trying to move away from drivers who I believe are dangerous. By profiling these drivers and intuitively rating them on a risk scale my decisions are impacted as are my route and speed. For instance, the distracted chatting woman and the aggressive young man were both profiled quickly as high risk because if the unexpected were to happen, I felt they would not be well-prepared to respond in a safe way so I changed lanes, altered speeds and moved away.

As parents of children with food allergies, I have learned that various people can be profiled to a certain extent when it comes to supervising my children with respect to their dairy and egg allergies. For instance, I've experienced an art teacher who gave my two-year-old egg-allergic-son an egg carton with which to create a craft, and when I pointed the problem out she said, *"Oh I didn't even think of that!"* I've also experienced another teacher who almost immediately forgot what foods my sons were allergic to right after our 20 minute meeting discussing it. Or there is the visitor who was just eating peanut butter candies in the car and has some smeared on their shirt. These 'non-registering/thinking' folks are profiled in my mind as the highest risk for food allergy supervision.

Another high risk category is for the people who act like parents of food allergic kids are a little crazy or at a minimum very over protective. For instance, one Sunday I came out of church service to find the Sunday school teacher gave the entire class sorbet and ice creams covered in chocolate sauce and other candies. Shocked, as I wasn't advised there would be sundaes in Sunday school, I inquired about the ingredients and mentally checked my purse for the Epi-Pen. The teacher's reaction was a bit condescending: I felt the strong sense that I was somehow stepping out of line. Even my mother advised me several years ago that my brother said if he watched the kids he wanted to try to give my sons some dairy! So I find these consciously rebellious attitudes as high risk profile, but perhaps not quite as high risk as the first category of, *"Geez, I forgot,"* or *"Geez, I didn't even think of that."* At least this second group is conscious.

On a positive note, there are wonderful low risk folks who are like angels. Both of my sisters-in-law and mother understand and go to special trouble to make delicious meals that are dairy and egg-free. I trust them, appreciate them and am grateful. Further, our new church's Sunday school teacher carefully explained her own experience and daughter's experience with food allergies all the while giving me assurances and food-related activity schedules so as to settle my own stomach.

So just like we profile others when driving or doing various every day activities that involve assessing risk, I think we can and should profile people upon whom we rely to care for or supervise our food-allergic children.

I think high risk personalities when it comes to food allergies people who tend to be absent minded, self-centered, forgetful, rebellious, arrogant and panicky. Their behavioral reputation will likely carry over to their ability to care for food-allergic children and either cause a crisis or be unlikely to handle a crisis well.

Look for people who show characteristics of being considerate, respectful and able to listen (and really hear what you are saying). Consider how carefully one communicates details. Do they have some experience with any serious health issue that might help them understand food allergies more? I think these are lower risk personalities and probably more likely to be successfully trusted to care for your food allergic child in a responsible, sensitive and positive way—both to your child and to you.

Roundtable Questions

1. Do you assess your friends and relatives according to how much you trust them with food allergies?

2. If you identify someone as 'high-risk' should you try to educate them or talk to them about your feelings?

3. Should you do something special to thank those people who 'get it' and go to special trouble to help you with the food allergies as social gatherings?

4. If a person is not trustworthy in other situations, should trust them in food allergy situations?

5. Should you try to change these people who you do not feel you can trust?

Parties

Whether it is a summer, school or birthday party it seems there is always food involved. Even after sporting events there is normally a snack. Over the past month, I've scampered to be ready for parties so that my kids don't feel left out and having something fun to eat. With all of these festivities for end of year, end of baseball season and beginning of summer, I had to add the food preparations reminders to my calendar just to keep it all straight.

There were only two unexpected incidents. One was good, the other was bad. Bad news first: We were at my older son's baseball game and snacks were being handed out which included fudgsicles and ice pops. My younger son wanted one. He is now seven and outgrew his dairy allergy at age five. But due to my older son's dairy allergy we still don't eat dairy so my younger son isn't used to it. Even so, I thought it would be alright for him to try the fudgsicle.

He took two licks and threw it away. Quickly he had a burning in his throat which led to his saying something was, "*In my throat.*" I am sure he was having a reaction. I gave him some antihistamine in the car on the way home and had the Epi-Pens ready. Once we were home, in less than five minutes, he was quite upset and it all seemed to be getting worse. There was no swelling of his face or lips, but he was crying and starting to panic. After a few more minutes his reaction subsided, but the whole thing was emotionally awful for all of us. We were worried, upset, even angry and of course my son was extremely scared. No more fudgsicles for us—but was dairy back off the table for my younger son? Had his dairy allergy returned?

Now the good news: About three days later, that same son had an end of year pizza party in his classroom. Knowing he never wanted to try the soy-based pizza we've had, I sent him in with a regular lunch of roast beef, carrots and other stuff. But he decided to try the dairy pizza that day. I found this out at dismissal and was shocked to learn that he had no reaction and that he actually liked the pizza!

So I am left wondering if it was something else in the fudgsicle that caused the reaction or if it was the difference between milk in the fudgsicle versus cheese on the pizza. Or was the difference caused by the dairy being cooked on the pizza as opposed to uncooked in the fudgsicle? I don't know. But I do know that despite the best of intentions and preparations, things happen at social gatherings, parties and celebrations. I am glad that I had my sons' medications with me and was ready to give it when needed.

Roundtable Questions

1. Should all sports, school or other impromptu parties be banned?

2. Could food at parties be banned or are we so oriented towards food that that is the main event?

3. Do you think it is sufficient to give those with food allergies special 'fun food' later if there is an unexpected party or no safe food at the party?

4. Should a parent ask what food will be at a party ahead of time?

5. Should event organizers be made aware that some kids have food allergies?

Holidays

Aren't the holidays are already hard enough? Seeing relatives who don't relate? Now add to that bowl of mixed nuts an allergy of tree nuts, peanuts or dairy allergy and there is likely to be an explosion of emotions. Take solace in the fact that firstly, you are not alone. Secondly, there are some ways to avoid the sparks—like the moms who have shared their stories in *Flourishing with Food Allergies*.

Here are some things to try:

- Two weeks before the holiday: Once you know who is hosting, you should start the communication by calling or emailing. Explain nicely something along the lines of, "*As you probably remember, our son/daughter is allergic to [nuts, peanuts, dairy, soy, egg] and so we want to make it easy for everyone involved so we will bring some allergy-free food for our child.*" This will take the pressure off of the hostess and also serve as a reminder to him or her when they are deciding on whether or not to buy a bag of tree nuts or peanuts for the coffee table. This may also allow the hostess to pass along the information to others who may be bringing food.

- One week before the holiday: Talk to your spouse and child in a formal way (i.e. at dinner or when there are limited distractions). Explain that you are going to Aunt Eat-A-Lot for Thanksgiving and you have contacted her to remind her of the allergy and advise her that you will be bringing some food for your son/daughter. If there is to be frustration expressed between spouses, it is best to air it well before the holiday and give it time to settle back down, rather than the night before or the day of the holiday. This communication will also set the expectation for your child that they will have their own food on the big day.

- One day before the holiday: Talk to your child again, alone and confirm what food they want at the big event. Tell them that you want to make them happy and have the foods they want. Make sure you have that food purchased, prepared and a ready-to-go-cooled container. Explain to your child that he or she is not allowed to eat *anything*, unless they ask you first. Tell them there will be many snacks that may make them sick. This way, your child has an expectation of the situation and will not be so angry to find out that they can't eat the food once they see it. Hopefully the fruit, vegetables and other some other safe snacks will make the child pleasantly surprised.

- On the holiday: Bring your child's requested, favorite foods as well as some traditional food for the holiday such as a turkey breast that you cooked or some corn bread that is safe. Most children don't like trying new foods so as long as their bellies and mouths are full with something they like, there will be fewer problems. By providing a new food or two (e.g. corn muffin, cranberry) their eyes and curiosity will hopefully be satisfied as well. Always remember to bring your child's Epi-Pen or Auvi-Q and some antihistamine with your own spoon or measuring cup.

At the holiday—try to relax. Keep an eye on your child without chasing them around. If there is an obvious problem with food placement (a plate of peanut butter cookies on the coffee table) casually move them to higher ground with a smile and some grace. Undoubtedly someone (often the less sensitive sorts) will try to engage in a food allergy discussion, often right in front of your children. Try to be nice and excuse yourself if you sense they are the disbelieving type and will try to argue about the reality of it. If the holiday environment is too chaotic or if you sense there will soon be a catastrophe, then keep it short and be on your way.

Keep your children safe and yourself calm.

Roundtable Questions

1. Should you simply not go to holiday events and dinners because of the food allergy?

2. Would you suggest specific foods to the host or do you think that would be rude?

3. Should you offer to bring a safe food or foods to share with others?

4. When a relative engages you in a food allergy conversation, when should you discuss it and when should you excuse yourself?

5. If your child or spouse complains about the allergy situation, should you take responsibility or ask them to take some actions such as making a safe food or talking with the host?

Family Feuds

Most of us want to partake in celebrations of Christmas, Hanukah, Easter, Halloween and other family and friend based traditions such as birthdays, graduations and other religious celebrations. From these events, we gather memories that carry us through our day-to-day lives and make us feel part of a bigger picture giving us a sense of belonging and happiness.

As expected, there is a lot of work for the host to prepare a gathering—food preparation often a large part. When food allergies enter the picture, then a level of stress can surround the event for both the parents and the host. If not addressed, this stress can erupt into anger, friction or even family fights. Don't let the event be ruined for you—there are things you can do so that your family can attend and do so safely. Attending these events is important for the social development of your child, as well as his or her happiness and emotional health, not to mention yours and your spouse's.

Unexpected, offending, allergen-laden foods can be a most difficult thing to handle. Here is a situation that caused one of the parents interviewed in *Flourishing with Food Allergies*, a great deal of frustration. "*Karen and her husband often have conflicting views on how to protect her son from an accidental ingestion of peanuts...Another example of contention is during the holiday season while at her mother-in-law's house one relative brought a plate of peanut butter cookies. Karen asked everyone not to eat them because the crumbs could fall to the floor and Max could ingest them. Rather than agreeing, her mother-in-law said, 'We'll just put them in the kitchen and eat them in there.' Karen was angry. Peanut could still fall to the floor in the kitchen, plus peanut traces would be on the fingers and lips of anyone who ate them and then might touch or kiss Max. She says, 'I felt unsupported by my husband as well because when I told him what his mother said, he didn't confront her [his mother].'*"

I think there are two main things you can do to ease the stress and plan for a relaxed and safer event. One of the things I have learned to do with my husband is to talk about the upcoming event as soon as I can. For instance, this past Thanksgiving we had plans to travel to my sister-in-law's house. She is quite aware of food allergies as her mother had celiac disease (intolerance to gluten) for a few years before her death. So, it is easy for me to communicate with her about the menu. She advised me what she was planning and I told her what I thought the boys would eat. We also decided what foods I would bring to allow safe and familiar foods for our boys. Together, we planned the meal over email about a week before the big day.

As soon as some of these details were worked out between my sister-in-law and me, I summarized them to my husband. I also advised him that I told her it was unnecessary for her to make all foods dairy-free, egg-free as she has offered to try to do in the past. Our boys are old enough (five and six) now to know they cannot just take whatever they want. I wanted my husband to be prepared when he saw the variety of foods on Thanksgiving Day. I also discussed the upcoming holiday with our sons and made sure to ask them what they really wanted to make their Thanksgiving Day special. In this case they wanted a homemade apple pie with some vanilla soy ice cream. So I advised my sister-in-law that I would also make and bring those for everyone to share.

Previously, I tried to *avoid* tension by waiting until that morning or the day before to discuss the event with my husband. This tended to not leave enough time for any concerns that he may have had and so I would find myself feeling annoyed that he had any concerns at all. Over the years, I have found that his concerns are reasonable and actually helpful. But again, to address these concerns in a relaxed way, i.e. to avoid stress and any conflict between us, there must be plenty of time between the initial discussion and the event, specifically at least a week. This leaves enough time to communicate again with the host or make a trip to the grocery store as needed, or even order something safe off of the Internet if I felt too busy to make it myself, like there are some dairy-free cookies I know I can get that are yummy and fun for the boys to open since each is individually wrapped. They are a little expensive, but sometimes it is worth it to avoid problems.

Another idea is to discuss other kinds of non-food related concerns that stem from the food allergy and can impact the situation. For example, I remember how important it was for me to feel that our boys did not feel different at birthday parties. Despite the fact that they had their own cupcakes, I wanted to give them those with ease, perhaps even laughter and lightheartedness at the party. I remember the tension I could feel emanating from my husband at a particular birthday party when we found that peanut butter and jelly sandwiches and cheese and crackers were being served. It was important for me that his tension didn't affect the children's enjoyment of the party.

Since I know my husband's mannerisms so well perhaps caused me to over react to his feelings—perhaps they were not noticeable to others, I do not know. At any rate, all went fairly smoothly, but I took something away from it.

I learned to discuss with him that I didn't want to feel tension nor did I want the boys to feel tension during the event. So well before the next event, I would say something along the lines of, "*I know how concerned you are about the boys coming into contact with allergy foods at parties. I am too,* (trying to show agreement) *but I also feel equally strong that it is important for the boys to not feel our tension at these gatherings.*" Then I'd be sure to listen to him. If he had specific concerns that I could address, I would do so, and get back to him as soon as I could.

I think this strategy can work for relatives as well. For instance, I have found that many people in the grandparent generation are so unfamiliar with the relatively new onslaught of serious food allergies in our children that they often find it unbelievable. Their beliefs then translate into actions, words, tones of voices, facial expressions, etc. that may cause us to feel that they think we are over reacting, are silly or are downright crazy. If possible, a parent might try to say something along these lines to the grandparent host of an upcoming event, "*I know that you feel Johnny's allergy might not be all that bad. But the doctor assures us that we should be very careful. My spouse and I would really appreciate it if you could not serve peanuts (or seafood or tree nuts, etc.) at your home that one day. We are really looking forward to the event. We just want to have a good time and not have to worry about Johnny. Is there anything I can do to help with organizing this?*"

For instance, you could specifically offer to contact the host's guests to request that they not bring foods that contain the allergy-ingredient. This might take the social burden and time burden off of the host. If you can get a list of phone numbers or email addresses, it may only take a short time to write a brief email explaining the allergy and how you'd appreciate it if people could help you in this way. I can't imagine that anyone would want to knowingly harm a child, so I am sure that most people will be happy to comply. But, not addressing this beforehand and waiting for the guest to arrive with dishes in hand, creates complications and hurt feelings with which no one wants to deal. Imagine Aunt Abby walks in with fifty dollars of shrimp cocktail only to find out that it will be put into the backroom. Or imagine Great Uncle Bob who spends hours making his famous peanut butter cookies the day before only to learn little Johnny is severely allergic.

There are many difficult tasks in the job of being a parent. Getting up at two o'clock in the morning for months on end is one of them! Caring and worrying over a child sick with a fever, cough or pneumonia is another. Even speaking up for the sake of your child when it feels uncomfortable and unnatural is also a difficult task. Know that you are not alone in the stress that you feel. Then, try to put a smile on your face and proactively talk to your spouse and relatives or friends well in advance (i.e. one or two weeks ahead of time) about the situation to address your concerns, their concerns and solutions. You can even pretend you are 'at work' if that's what it takes to remain nice and calm. It will make the event much better for your child, you, your spouse, the host and the other guests.

Roundtable Questions

1. Have you ever tried to discuss the food allergies with a host before an event, how did it turn out?

2. What is the biggest problem that you have with your spouse and children when attending these events?

3. How do you feel about approaching other people about the allergy? Does it make you nervous or angry?

4. Have you ever asked someone to put away food that is not safe for your children?

5. Do you think you leave a party once you arrive and determine that is simply too unsafe?

Summertime

As the end of the school year approaches, there are new situations, parties and trips coming up for the next three months. How can we have fun while keeping our food-allergic children safe? We don't want to miss out, nor should our children miss out on all the fun.

Here are a few tips:

1. <u>Never forget the Auvi-Q or Epi-Pens:</u> Remember not to leave it in the hot car. The ideal temperature if 77ºF but it can withstand the range of about 60ºF to 85ºF. If we are going out for the day and packing a cooler, I will put the epinephrine in the outer pocket of the cooler—i.e. not too cold but a bit more stable than my purse.

2. <u>Always bring safe food for your child:</u> You want to relax and have fun too, right? Do not interpret that as 'loosening up' and letting your child eat foods that may not be safe. I made this mistake once—at a BBQ I let my son have a hot dog roll without checking the ingredients. It turned out that the bun had butter and milk in it. My son developed a mild reaction of coughing due to the mucus. We gave him an antihistamine and it was gone within 20 minutes.

3. <u>Remember the antihistamine:</u> You can purchase the single dose tablets or liquid spoon servings and put some in the epinephrine case. This way you don't need to remember two items—just bring the single item that contains both epinephrine and antihistamine. Go to the trouble to buy a little case at the store (I like camera cases at the office supply store) that will properly fit everything you need including any other medications the child may need like an inhaler.

Summer fun is more fun when you are responsible. That's when you can really relax because you have all of the bases covered.

Roundtable Questions

1. If you forget the epinephrine (Auvi-Q or Epi-Pen) should you go back and get it? If so, how far would you travel back?

2. If you forget the antihistamine should you go back and get it or stop to buy some?

3. If you forget to bring safe food, would you stop to buy some or take a chance at the party?

4. Is it more relaxing to be at a party having made all the preparations or is it too much work to bring all those items?

5. Should we simply avoid parties so that our children are not made to feel different?

Dining Out

Are you or your child scared to eat outside of your home? Do you wonder exactly what is in food that has been prepared by a friend or a restaurant? Do you trust the person who made it? Do you trust the waiter who explains what is in it? Do they know the seriousness of your food allergy?

Not only is it perfectly natural to feel apprehensive about eating a food that is prepared without the mandated regulations that help to define ingredient lists and methods for food preparation, but I think it is smart as well. For instance, my mother is allergic to MSG and develops migraine headaches when she has some. She often asks wait staff whether the soup, gravy or dressing contains it—but she is often suspicious when the reply is too quickly, *"Oh no—none of that."* To make matters more complex, MSG is often hidden by other names such as 'hydrolyzed vegetable protein' she researched in Dr. George Schwartz's book, *The MSG Syndrome*.

Another example of caution is our friend's daughter--who has allergies to peanuts and tree nuts. She comes to my son's birthday parties year after year—her parents are so much fun. While her mom checks with me about the ingredients in the cupcakes or cake and I advise her there are no peanuts, tree nuts, dairy or egg her daughter usually opts for her own home-baked cupcake. Why? She feels safer and so the party is more fun and relaxing for her.

A hostess should never ever feel insulted or not trusted if a food-allergic person doesn't eat food they prepared, even if the hostess went to trouble to make it allergen-free. Consider cross contamination that can easily occur. Perhaps yesterday a peanut butter and jelly sandwich was made on a cutting board. That night it was washed, but there are protein residues remaining in the board. Then vegetable or fruit is sliced and picks up those peanut proteins—this can easily affect a child or adult with a peanut allergy. A hostess should also consider the consequences of a mistake. We all make mistakes. Do we want to be responsible for making a mistake that can actually cause someone to have to go to the hospital? I think not.

We really don't know what it is like to have a food allergy, unless we have one. I have tried, many a time, to imagine what it would be like to have a food allergy myself, but I probably just can't get there one hundred percent. I know what is it like to have children with life threatening food allergies—it makes a mother worry—really worry, to say the very least.

The best thing a hostess can do when having food allergic guests is to: (a) Not get insulted if they bring their own food or refuse something even if the hostess went to some trouble to make it allergy-free; and (b) Save the packages of store bought food so that the food allergic person (or parent) can double-check the ingredients to ensure there are no allergens—or produced in a factory where allergens exist. I have heard of children reacting to cookies made in a factory that also handles peanut containing foods, for instance. It is no joke.

The bottom line is that children, adults and parents should feel perfectly justified in doing what makes them and their children safe. Hosts should be understanding—even if they can't completely appreciate what it feels like to have a food allergy or what can happen to a person if they ingest the allergen. Be nice.

Roundtable Questions

1. Should you take your food allergic child to restaurants?

2. Should you trust homemade foods if the person assures you that the food is allergen-free?

3. Should you provide ingredients lists to guests who are coming to your party?

4. If you go to a lot of trouble to make allergen-free food, and the child refuses it, what would you do?

5. Have you ever experienced someone getting annoyed or insulted over food allergy ingredient questions?

Trips and Travel

Last week we took our first big family vacation to Disney and Sea World. Our boys are eight and nine and we waited until now for several reasons. First, we wanted them to remember it. I only vaguely remember my childhood trip when I was five. My husband has advised that the cognitive memory doesn't develop until after five. Second, we were concerned about our kids' food allergies to dairy and egg. Waiting until these ages has helped because our younger son outgrew his dairy allergy at age five and his egg yolk allergy at age seven. Now we only need to contend with his egg white allergy and our older son's dairy and egg allergy—which are now moderate, no longer severe. Furthermore, the boys want to eat foods that do not make them sick.

We decided to stay in a resort off-site so that we could have a little extra room and a full kitchen. My mother was kind enough to purchase some allergen-free groceries for us and bring them to our room. We cooked and ate in our room whenever we could. This served us well—as we were comfortable with the foods we were eating and it kept the costs down as compared to dining in a restaurant for every meal. My friend advised me that she used Green Grocer to order food and have it delivered to their room. She advised that it was a little more expensive than a normal grocery store—but still, probably less than dining out or renting a car to do the grocery shopping.

When we could not eat in our room because we were on-site at Disney and Sea World, we learned the protocol for ordering allergen-free foods. In both places, we were required to order through a manager. The manager had the ingredients of each food and was able to show it to us. Disney seemed more prepared to do this, with ingredient lists in a ready-prepared-binder, while Sea World had to bring out the bag of the item. Disney assured us that the foods would be prepared in a kitchen that was set up for allergy-folk and even had a separate fryer for foods like French fries to avoid cross contamination. Sea World had a separate grill for cooking burgers, chicken and assured us they used a separate fryer as well for French fries. Both places provided us with foods that our kids could eat without any allergic reactions—but we felt safer with the Disney restaurant. They seemed to be more educated and prepared for the food-allergy parent.

One final word—we took a day off in between each day at the parks. Our sons (and we) needed the rest and I think it served us all well. As we all know, kids who have food allergies are dealing with an immune system that is over-reactive. So I think it is important to not stress those kids' bodies too much—such as taking them to a theme park every day for several days in a row. Be sure to read the theme park's literature on food allergies before you go, so that you feel prepared.

Roundtable Questions

1. Do you feel so worried about food allergies that you avoid travelling?

2. Should theme parks cater to people who have food allergies? If so, how?

3. Is getting a hotel room with a kitchen a good option for those with food allergies?

4. Have you had a good or bad experience with travelling while having food allergies?

5. Should airlines offer more accommodations for those with food allergies? Should they carry epinephrine?

Medical Topics

New Physicians

This past year we switched our health insurance carrier. Now we have to switch our doctors as well. New doctors have new ideas, beliefs and strategies. I am trying to keep an open mind without becoming too hopeful or doubtful. After having gone on the emotional roller coaster every year for the past nine years, I now try to stabilize myself. Even so, I do find the depth of my feelings about my oldest son's food allergies sneak up like an earthquake while talking to the doctors.

Our new allergist thinks that our younger son, who is now nine years old, is ready for a challenge test for cooked egg. So I am to scramble an egg (do I remember how to do this?) and bring it to the office in a few weeks for his challenge test.

The allergist is also optimistic about our older son's allergies, now that he is ten years old, after seeing the blood test results from one year ago. She thinks that they are not as severe as we've been told. It is frustrating to me that the results are confusing—our test shows a scale of 1 to 5 he is moderate for milk and high for egg. The numbers on the scale correlate to more numbers: Low being in the less than one (in a decimal range) and very high being close to 100. The scale seems to be one that rises exponentially, so our high is in the 5 range, but the very high runs from 17 to over 100. I've further been advised that depending upon the situation, these numbers can all be quite meaningless. For instance, if your child's toxic load (due to stress, pollen, etc.) is high, then his or her reaction can be higher than expected to the allergen based upon the test results alone. Nothing seems concrete or reliable.

So maybe our new allergist's approach will be helpful. She wants me to boil milk five times over and bring that cooked milk, along with regular milk and the scrambled egg for a skin prick test for our older son. So rather than using the lab created food allergens, we'll just use the real thing. We'll see how it goes in a couple of weeks and I'll try not to get on that emotional roller coaster. But *that* is almost impossible.

Roundtable Questions

1. Have you switched doctors and if so, for what reason?

2. When you see different doctors, do you get different guidance?

3. Do you feel like you are on an emotional roller coaster when you visit the allergist?

4. Does your allergist offer any counseling or are they more matter of fact?

5. How can you improve your emotional state and your child's before and after a visit?

Physician Likability

Today we went to our regular pediatrician for my older son's nine year old checkup. Our pediatrician is an allopathic doctor who prescribes all of the regular medications, vaccinations and tracks my son's growth in height and weight. But he does more than that—which is why I like him. He talks to us and listens with an open mind. He values learning— not just teaching me, but learning from us as well.

Just over three years ago, I began bringing our son to a naturopath physician. This was something new for us and seemed very different if not questionable. My husband was skeptical and gave a timeline of three months for some improvement to occur—which it did. Our son's long standing sinus problems were healed by this route.

Not only did my husband maintain an open mind, but our doctor, the allopathic pediatrician, did as well. Since then, over the past three years, I have kept our pediatrician in the loop on our efforts to improve our older son's health and both of our sons' chances for outgrowing their food allergies. Our pediatrician has never once shown to be anything less than fully open minded about the situation. He has told us that although this is not his area of expertise, he is interested in what supplements or herbs our sons are being given. He is also interested and makes copies of any test results that are run by the naturopath doctor. I respect his behavior and attitude immensely—and am grateful that I have such an intelligent and open minded doctor who tries to maintain a balance. He listens and then adds value by explaining his perspective.

During my son's exam, we found that he cannot see very well. This is no surprise to me, as my own eyesight requires correction and has since I was about nine years old as well. While I had taken my son to an optometrist last summer, we find the reading glasses he was prescribed really are insufficient for his distance learning. So my pediatrician said to me, *"Just like you researched food allergies to find solutions that work for you, don't be hesitant about finding an eye doctor that works for your son. Get a second opinion. Or even a third. If insurance doesn't cover it, just pay for it."* Wow—how many doctors are that honest?

Another similar thing happened before our appointment this morning, when we were at swim team practice. While I sat on the bleachers chatting with a mom who I respect she explained her feelings to me about her latest appointment with an allergist. She told me about the condescension, out-of-date medication prescribed and difference of opinion about necessity of certain medicines and medicine-based tests. Having gone to this same allergist last summer, I recalled how uncomfortable I felt with the asthma test they gave my son last year because it required a few doses of medication even though he didn't need it. I remember the allergist implying that I was wrong not to give my son any dairy or egg. But then she completely changed her mind once she witnessed his skin prick test results. I also recalled the feeling I had while leaving that office—like cattle being moved slowly through a painful livestock route. I felt frustrated, tired and angry.

When I came home today after our swim team practice and our pediatrician appointment, I switched this year's upcoming allergy appointment to our original small town allergist who has given us honest advice such as—avoid peanuts and other highly allergic foods until our sons outgrow the dairy and egg allergies. I also switched our eye doctor to a new doctor recommended by the pediatrician. I feel better already. Remember, your mind, your child, your insurance, your money are under your control and choice.

Roundtable Questions

1. Do you like your doctor? Pediatrician? Allergist? Others?

2. Do any of them make you feel like you are less than them, inferior or not smart?

3. Does your doctor listen with an open mind?

4. When your doctor responds, is it fast or do they take at least a few seconds to consider what you have said and your unique situation?

5. How do you feel when leaving your doctor's office? Better or angry?

Physicians, Nurses and Tests

My kids are still young, ages five and six, as of this writing. Even so we've been through our fair share of allergy tests. My boys have each had several skin prick tests and one blood test each. One son has had a challenge test and the other is currently scheduled for one.

At the last blood test, the blood-taking nurse said to my five year old, "So you don't feel so good after eating certain foods, huh?" Then she laughed heartily. I was dumbfounded. I think my five year old was too. I sat on the chair holding him on my lap and we said nothing. We just looked at her back as she had turned around after laughing to enter a few items into her computer. How could a nurse or anyone be so insensitive as to ask a question like that when she knows he has food allergies and then laugh out loud? What was she laughing at? Our misfortune? If she wasn't about to take three little vials of blood from my 'baby' I might have just confronted her on why she was laughing.

Aside from the lack of personal tact, there are other frustrations that I have with food allergy testing. Specifically, skin prick tests can show false positives, meaning it may show that you are allergic to X when in fact you are not. Further, the blood tests can show false negatives, meaning it may show you are *not* allergic to Y when in fact you are. Then there is the ultimate 'challenge' test where you child eats or drinks the food in a substantial quantity, which you have studiously avoided for the past few years.

When my older son went in for his dairy challenge test, his blood test had been negative but the skin prick was positive. The doctor said he was, "*90% sure he would not react during the challenge test to the dairy.*" But, he *did* react and had to receive epinephrine in the doctor's office. Our current allergist advised us that she would only do a challenge test if *both* the skin prick and blood tests come back negative. This seems to make more sense to me so we are on our path to this test now.

Roundtable Questions

1. Have you experienced an insensitive nurse, doctor or testing situation? If so, what did you do?

2. How do you feel about your allergist's testing approach?

3. Do the blood test and skin prick test leave you with more questions than answers?

4. Which type of test do you trust most: Skin, blood or challenge?

5. Do you think there should be a better way to test for food allergies and if so how can we get there?

Food Allergy Testing

It has been my experience that food allergy tests can be a bit unreliable. It is best to use combinations of allergy tests to get the most accurate readings and results. Normally you will have to ask your child's allergist to do more than one type of test. You can even request that your doctor order the results to be sent to more than one lab for more accurate readings. Further, consider getting a second opinion from a different allergist.

Sounds like a lot of work? Perhaps. But consider the impact of food allergies on your life and your child's life. Eliminating a single food from your child's or family's diet can be a lot more work and for a much longer time. It can also contribute to stress in your life and in your child's life because it affects both social life and school life. When food allergy testing normally comes around every year or two, it isn't unreasonable to make sure the results are really accurate since you'll have to live with them for a long time.

The following is a summary of food allergy tests that you can seek out for your child. Due to the rate of inaccuracy from single tests, combining results can give you a clearer picture of your child's situation. Because different labs and doctors can produce different results from the same tests, don't be shy about getting a second opinion. Call your insurance company about coverage for additional tests. Share the test results with all the doctors involved to they can learn as well. Any doctor who gets annoyed that you have asked for a second opinion does not have your child's health concerns first.

- Skin prick tests: This involves pricking the skin with various allergens. The benefit of this type of test is that it will probably not give a false negative meaning if the child has an allergy—it will appear. But the con is that it can give a false positive meaning that it may show an allergy when in fact the child can tolerate the food.

- Blood tests: Several types exist such as the RAST (Radioallergosorbent Test) and ELISA (enzyme-linked immunosorbent assay). The results can be misleading in that sometimes the child will be allergic to the food but the test will result in a negative result. The blood taken from the child's arm can be split and sent to two different labs for more accurate results. You will need to request that this be done.

- Kinesiology tests: This is done by homeopathic physicians using a small vile of the allergen which is held in the hand of a patient while muscle strength is tested. It is a non-invasive non-painful test and easy to do—but the subjective and interpretive nature of the results may put some people off as to its validity.

- Challenge tests: This test involves eating the offending allergy-food in the doctors' office. It is normally recommended when BOTH blood and skin prick tests are negative. It is a lengthy test (3-4 hours most of which is waiting) and is normally done when there is a very good chance the child has outgrown the food allergy.

- New tests in the future: *"A new kind of blood test could someday help doctors zero in more definitively on who is most likely to have allergic reaction to foods. Phadia AB, a maker of allergy tests, has developed a test, called Component-Resolved Diagnostis (CRD) that can determine which molecule within a food is sparking the antibody reaction. In the peanut, for example, only three of 14 different molecules are associated with anaphylaxis-causing reaction, according to the company. CRD has not yet been submitted for approval by the Food and Drug Administration, but it is in use in Europe…In the Manchester study, for example, the researchers found that almost all of the children who were highly allergic to peanuts reacted to a specific protein call Ara h 2…Knowing more about what specific molecules cause allergic reactions could help scientists understand more about the severity of allergic reactions, and someday help efforts to develop treatments to trick the immune system into behaving differently."*[14]

- Delayed allergy tests: Most allergy testing is for immediate allergies (with symptoms of hives, anaphylaxis, vomiting, breathing, swelling, rashes, eczema). But for many the symptoms are not so obvious—making the connection between cause and symptom downright difficult. Delayed food allergies can be tested for through blood testing (only) as described above. But instead of searching for IgE antibodies, the lab must look for IgG or IgA antibodies. You will need to find an allergist who is knowledgeable in this area. Parents and children dealing with asthma, autism and ADHD often have delayed food allergy antibodies. Be careful though as your insurance may not cover this type of test.

In summary, take your child to an allergist for allergy testing. Ask for more than one kind of test and consider getting a second opinion. Share results among the doctors and labs. Understand that immediate allergies are different from delayed allergies, but both can affect a child's life drastically.

Roundtable Questions

1. What different types of allergy tests have you or your child taken?

2. Do you have any idea where the results are being sent or if there are differences in the labs?

3. Have you heard of delayed allergies? Do you believe they can impact a child's health and behavior?

4. What do you think of homeopathy or naturopathy? Do you think it could help your child or is it too different to consider?

5. Do you think the government or someone should invest more funding into better food allergy tests?

Second Opinions

Getting a second opinion from medical professionals can benefit all sorts of medical conditions—not just allergies. Will it cost a little more money? Maybe a few extra co-pays, but in the long run, I think it is better.

For instance, my sons now have three kinds of doctors: A regular, allopathic pediatrician, a pediatric allergist and a naturopathic physician.

1. The allopathic pediatrician tends to give vaccinations, run annual weight and measurement checks and prescribe medications such as antibiotics and other strong, immediate-response medicines;

2. The pediatric allergist will run allergy skin prick tests, blood tests when necessary and challenge tests when both of the former are negative. The allergist is also focused what medications might help avoid seasonal allergies from growing into illness and what medications are need for severe allergic reactions such as an epinephrine; and

3. The naturopathic physician is a fully licensed doctor with as many years of schooling as a regular doctor. But the focus here is on the person's health as a whole and to identify what might be missing from a person's body that is causing illness or other problems. Then the solution is giving or supplementing the missing resource to allow the person to heal their own body, perhaps more slowly but also more fully.

Often the doctors have different opinions about how to handle our sons' illnesses which can be confusing and frustrating. Other times, I appreciate the two-against-one sort of outcome because it helps me to see the situation more clearly by separating out the different doctors' methodologies and focus.

Here's an example: Last spring seasonal pollen was very high. My son was wheezing. I took him to the naturopath and then the allopathic doctor in the same day. The naturopath gave him some supplements to help his breathing and suggested the situation warranted a breathing treatment inhalant. Because he isn't licensed to prescribe that type of medication he wanted me to see the allopathic physician, right away. Once I was at the next office, the allopathic physician thought my son needed not only the breathing treatment inhalant, but also steroids and antibiotics. Later, at home when I called and advised the naturopath physician of this solution, he disagreed, but left it to my discretion. I gave my son the inhalant for one week and the steroids because it seemed like he needed them to get over this wheezing problem. But I didn't give him the antibiotics because he didn't have a fever so I thought he didn't have a sinus infection. It turned out that he was fine without the antibiotics.

Here's where the second and third opinion helped: The allopathic (regular pediatric) physician said there was nothing wrong with steroids for a few days. But there *was* an impact that has lasted for over four months. My son developed a rash from the steroids that we gave him for just a few days. Beating down the rash with months of probiotics wasn't working. It was not until I bought several over the counter creams, washes and powders to kill off the candida fungus did the rash start to subside. I also wonder what other negative impacts occurred that are invisible to me.

While the naturopath said the steroids caused the rash problem by empowering bad bacteria and fungus in my son's system, I also heard the pediatrician say they wouldn't cause any problems if only taken for a few days and he didn't think the rash was due to the steroids (even though it appeared soon after taking them). But then the scales tipped for me when the pediatric allergist said that we should avoid oral steroids. A preventative seasonal allergy medication is worth taking to avoid the onset of wheezing and thus the need for steroids. I think the problem with steroids is that they do throw the body's balance off which is not something a parent wants for a child who has food allergies since the delicate balance of intestinal health is probably the source of the problem in the first place.

Sometimes I feel frustrated by one doctor or another. But I also really like each of my sons' doctors as kind, thoughtful, educated persons. I do believe they all mean well and only want to do the best for my children. So I will continue to obtain doctors' advice and opinions as each has different personalities, educations, philosophies about the right way to treat and heal.

I think one of the most difficult parts of being a parent involves weighing the information and making an informed decision. How could I be fully informed if I only had a single professional opinion?

Getting second and third opinions is a good thing. Maybe it is more complex, but it is more complete.

Roundtable Questions

1. How many doctors do you or your child visit?

2. Do you share opinions of doctors with one another?

3. If there is a conflicting opinion between doctors, how do you decide what to do?

4. What are some of the key factors in how you approach your child's or your health? Based upon values?

5. If there is a conflict, do you feel pressured by one doctor's opinion? Is it due to fear? Or social pressure?

Treatments

There is a commercial on television that really upsets my eight year old. The image is of a mother holding her baby while she is coughing. My son started yelling, *"Why is she holding him if she has a cough!"* He was definitely taken in by that contagious situation portrayed in the commercial. The advertiser wants to frighten the viewer into getting a vaccination so that we don't pass on whooping cough to our child (they also want to increase sales of their vaccination).

My older ten year old son was watching a different commercial on play dough. He saw a new toy that can be used to mix the dough into various shapes. Then he adeptly realized that that will ruin the play dough and will cause the kids to need to buy more. I was amazed that he figured that out and further said that it was probably the strategy of the company to increase their sales, not only through the toy, but also for more dough.

Soon after these incidents, I received an email from an allergy mom web site. She appeared to be promoting a new drug to cure allergies. I looked up the drug on the Internet and did some superficial research. The drug Omalizumab sold under the name of Xolair appears to help those with allergies within a relatively short period of time. When I reviewed the side effects, there was some discussion of cancer—but no overwhelming proof that this drug caused cancer but some evidence such as, *"This medicine may increase your risk of certain types of cancer[15]"* and *"Oncologic side effects have included malignancies in 0.5% of patients (n=4127) compared with 0.2% of control patients (n=2236). The types of malignancies in omalizumab-treated patients included breast, skin (nonmelanoma), prostate, melanoma, and parotid."*[16] No thanks—I'd prefer not to have to deal with another serious problem.

All of this reminded me of when a company had approached me, soon after my first book was published, to develop a food allergy web site with them. Their primary goal was to 'monetize' the sight. This meant they would add advertisements and links to products that would generate hits and money for my site. I declined. My primary objective in writing my book and blog was and still is to reach out and help others, not to profit.

When a person's goals get confused, so do their values and thus their actions. For example, once income is the primary goal, then other values can become compromised. I had this impression from this aforementioned allergy web site years ago. The articles in each newsletter contained a lot of links to products and their web sites. Was the founder of this site recommending all of these products or just trying to generate income from them? I think that site is an example of a highly monetized enterprise. The bottom line is that we as consumers and parents of children with food allergies need to be a somewhat skeptical or at least be inquisitive.

The term 'Buyer Beware' is explained as, *"A warning that notifies a buyer that the goods he or she is buying are 'as is,' or subject to all defects. When a sale is subject to this warning the purchaser assumes the risk that the product might be either defective or unsuitable to his or her needs. This rule is not designed to shield sellers who engage in fraud or bad faith dealing by making false or misleading representations about the quality or condition of a particular product. It merely summarizes the concept that a purchaser must examine, judge, and test a product considered for purchase by him or herself."*[17]

My purpose in this topic and recommendation is to take a good look at drugs and do your own research on allergy related products. Consider who is recommending them and why? Are they getting a kick-back for the sale of this product? Are there negative side effects of this product that you are willing to accept for your child? How long has the product been on the market? How many studies have been done? Are there alternative products that may not be heavily marketed because there is no large company behind them to generate a profit?

Consider your options carefully and fully.

Roundtable Questions

1. When you read an advertisement or a web site are you excited about new products or skeptical?

2. Do you jot down the name of the product or drug and research it or rely only a doctor's opinion?

3. What kinds of drugs do you and your children take and what are the side effects?

4. If there are some dangerous side effects, when do you think it worth the risk?

5. Do you ever consider natural solutions, i.e. diet related solutions, like cilantro for eliminating mercury?

Desensitization or Avoidance

Our youngest son who turned nine in August has just outgrown his egg allergy. Last year his skin prick test to egg white was negative, but it was a one or two to the egg yolk. So this year, our new allergist wanted to try a challenge test where he ate some egg. So I scrambled up an egg and we went down to the doctor's where they gave him a tiny bit of egg in increasing amounts over an hour or so. He had no reaction at all so we were pleased. Our strategy had been strict avoidance of egg over the past nine years of his life, which wasn't difficult for us because his older brother is allergic to egg and dairy.

Our happiness at this last allergy appointment was mitigated somewhat by our older son's test results. He did not have a challenge test—only a skin prick test. His allergies are to egg and dairy. Both of these results showed a highly positive response. So while we've been careful to avoid egg and dairy, that avoidance has worked for one son but not for the other. The boys are physically different—maybe this plays into it.

We will continue with our dairy drops for our older son. Thankfully our new allergist thinks that this is a good approach for slowly and carefully desensitizing our son to his allergies without any risk. This works well with our homeopathic doctor's philosophy too. I've noticed there are a lot more homeopathic drops on the market now than there were even a few years ago, when I was researching desensitization.

So we will continue, but with the satisfaction that our younger son is now out-of-the-woods, so to speak.

Roundtable Questions

1. Do you think that desensitization through oral drops or baked foods works?

2. Do you think it is dangerous? When would you not want to try it?

3. Does avoidance of foods work to heal an allergy by allowing the IgE antibody to disintegrate?

4. Should parents be aggressive in finding solutions to their children's allergies even if it means including some drug related options?

5. How do you feel about homeopathic approaches that attempt to heal the whole body, which in turn should heal the problems stemming from the base issues?

Desensitization Techniques

A few weeks ago, my nine year old son was eating lunch at school when his little buddy dipped his carrot in ranch dressing and touched my son's cheek with it. My friend who works at the school saw my son scratching two red bumps on his face and she immediately guessed that somehow he came into contact with an allergen. She sent him to the nurse who gave him some antihistamine which worked to calm the hives within a short time—but my son was shaken, upset and wanted to go home.

While he has never had a reaction to merely touching dairy—he had now. Rather than becoming less sensitive, it appears he may be becoming more sensitive. Have our efforts of strict avoidance backfired on us? I don't have the answers, but did some research on how we might approach desensitizing him.

I found four main approaches:

1. New Drug 'Omalizumab': *"'This is the first study to use omalizumab in combination with oral desensitization,' said Umetsu, who is also the Prince Turki bin Abdul Aziz al-Saud Professor of Pediatrics at Harvard Medical School. 'Using omalizumab allowed us to escalate their milk intake very rapidly compared to other desensitization protocols, and still limit allergic reactions.' After first pretreating the children with omalizumab, the investigators then introduced milk in ever-increasing amounts over the next seven to 10 weeks, a relatively rapid desensitization period."*[18]

2. Hospitalized with Antihistamine & Epinephrine: *"The treatment consists of progressive oral administrations of the allergen, starting with infinitesimal quantities and increasing the dose every two hours (5 to 3 doses daily). Antihistamine is given twice a day, and an IV catheter is maintained on the patient for the duration of the treatment, so that adrenaline can be administered without delay in case of an emergency. The treatment lasts about 10-12 days, and is later continued at home following a sequence determined by the hospital."*[19]

3. Baked Milk: *"Dr. Anna Nowak-Wegrzyn , 'Our unpublished data (in older kids, median age about 4 years; Caubet JC et al, manuscript under revision) suggested that casein-IgE <0.7 kUA/L is a very favorable prognostic factor for tolerance of*

baked milk with the vast majority of kids tolerating baked milk with such level."[20]

4. Homeopath Desensitization: "*The term homeopathy comes from the Greek words homeo, meaning similar, and pathos, meaning suffering or disease. Homeopathy seeks to stimulate the body's ability to heal itself by giving very small doses of highly diluted substances. According to the 2007 National Health Interview Survey, which included a comprehensive survey of complementary and alternative medicine...('CAM') use[d] by Americans, an estimated 3.9 million U.S. adults and approximately 900,000 children used homeopathy in the previous year. People use homeopathy for a range of health concerns, from wellness and prevention, to the treatment of diseases and conditions such as allergies, asthma, chronic fatigue syndrome, depression, digestive disorders, ear infections, headaches, and skin rashes.*"[21]

Roundtable Questions

1. Would you consider taking a more aggressive approach to desensitization and if so which appeal to you?

2. Would you pay for hospitalization out of pocket if insurance didn't cover it to attempt to cure allergies?

3. Do you think desensitization is risky and that it would be safer to wait until the body heals itself?

4. When would you change your mind from you current belief? What would a threshold be?

5. Has strict avoidance worked for you or anyone you know?

Oral Immunization Therapy

OIT is Oral Immunotherapy—according to Brian P. Vickery, MD, instructor for the department of pediatrics in the division of pediatric allergy and immunology at Duke University School of Medicine—it is a process of, *"the careful daily administration of gradually increasing doses of allergen...[that can modify] the allergic immune response, and the amount of allergen required to cause a reaction is increased to levels well above those which would be expected in an accidental ingestion."*[22] This procedure should not be undertaken at home and is still in its experimental stages.

The process is currently under investigation and study. Based upon my reading and understanding of Dr. Nowak-Wegrzyn's opinion in *Allergy and Clinical Immunology*, some of the considerations are: (1) Whether the long term impact and possible benefits of giving OIT outweigh the long term benefits of totally avoiding the allergic-food in hopes that the body will naturally develop a tolerance to it; (2) the possibly dangerous side effects of using OIT to try to develop a tolerance to the allergy-food because there may be allergic reactions during this process; and (3) factors to deal with during the process that may make it unpredictable such as variables that may affect treatment tolerance like illness, exercise, dosing on an empty stomach and asthma. The researchers appear to state that it is too soon to draw conclusions as to whether the short term benefits OIT outweigh the risks associated with it and the hope that long term food avoidance may be a more solid solution.[23]

As a mother of six and seven year old boys who are allergic to egg and egg/dairy respectively, I continue to be interested in this therapy. But, both our pediatric allergist and naturopathic physician concur that until our older son outgrows his seasonal environmental allergies that manifest in itchy eyes, sneezing and perhaps a slight cough, we should not attempt any food allergy drops. Hopefully we will get to the point where either they both outgrow their food allergies naturally through our avoidance practices or the studies advance to the point where everyone involved (physicians, my husband and me, and our sons) feel okay about trying one of these proactive therapies. Until then we will watch and wait.

Roundtable Questions

1. Do you know if prepared drops are offered on the market for your or your child's allergy?

2. If there are no prepared drops could your doctor make some for you?

3. Do you consider this to be a viable solution to desensitizing a seriously allergic person?

4. At what age do you think this type of therapy could be safely provided to a child?

5. How long do you think it would or should take for this type of therapy to have an impact?

Controversial Topics

Pregnancy

When I was pregnant with my first son I didn't even think about food allergies. I worried about just about everything else—spinobifida, Downs and about one hundred other problems that I read about—but not food allergies. I tried to drink milk because I heard it was good (no doubt from dairy industry advertising). I ate peanut butter and jelly crackers as I did throughout my life for an evening snack or occasional lunch. Oddly I craved eggs, especially during the first trimester for each of my sons. Both of my sons remain allergic to eggs now at ages 5 and 7. Only one remains allergic to dairy—the oldest. We are seem to be okay with peanuts and tree nuts (almonds, beechnuts, Brazil nuts, cashews, chestnuts, gingko, hazelnuts, hickory nuts, macadamia nuts, pecans, pine nuts, pistachios and walnuts) as we have avoided them.

In retrospect, had I known that my own family history showed a strong tendency towards dairy and egg allergies and if I had been more informed about food allergies in general, perhaps I would have avoided eating these foods while I was pregnant. My cousin and his father, my uncle, both had egg and dairy allergies when they were infants. My cousin even had to be hospitalized during his third month of life for lack of weight gain. My aunt told me that she had to feed him soy formula after that occasion. Now my cousin is in his late thirties and he still avoids milk but that it is not life threatening to him—only sickening.

If I were pregnant again, I'd might eat what I eat now—a dairy and egg-free diet. I rarely eat peanuts and tree nuts since after seven years of not eating I find them difficult to digest. My diet is focused on potatoes, rice, meat, fish and lots of vegetables and fruit. I think that is a good diet for pregnancy, unless there is a history of a fish or shellfish allergy, at which point I'd avoid that as well. Normally food allergies develop for high protein foods because the body can have trouble properly digesting those foods. The big eight are: soy, wheat, egg, dairy, fish, shellfish, peanut and tree nuts.

Another action that I would take would be to supplement myself with probiotics. Probiotics are good bacteria that can rebalance a person's intestinal tract so that it can properly digest foods. If a person's intestinal tract is damaged by overuse of antibiotics, then the food can go into the blood stream through little holes in the intestinal wall—a disorder known as 'leaky gut syndrome.' There have been some studies that show that pregnant women who supplement with probiotics have a lower incidence of having babies with food allergies, as detailed in my first book's probiotics chapter. Even supplementing after the child is born, if the mother is breastfeeding, can help the baby avoid food allergies.

Recently, I read a book called *Hidden Food Allergies,* by James Braley and Patrick Holford. It is the first time that I have seen a recommendation by a doctor along this line. The book states, *"Pregnant women who suffer from allergies have been found to be more likely to have babies who develop allergies and asthma, according to a five-year study funded by the British Lung Foundation and Asthma U.K. The researchers, however, found that it is possible to minimize that risk by reducing a woman's exposure to allergens while she is pregnant. Dr. Jill Warner said, our research shows that mothers can influence whether their baby develops sensitization to allergies. Controlling the mothers' reactions to allergens, especially during the second and third trimesters of pregnancy, may well be the treatment of the future."*[24]

In summary, avoiding known family allergens and common allergens (like peanuts or the other big eight listed above) while supplementing with probiotics during pregnancy and breastfeeding months can help a mother ward off allergies in her baby. It may be too early to prove this through studies and there can be conflicting viewpoints. Personally, we were told to wait to introduce peanuts to our boys until they outgrew their allergies. Once our younger son outgrew his dairy allergy, we tried one half of a raw, organic peanut several times over a few weeks (dry roasted peanuts can cause more allergies than boiled or raw peanuts). He had no reaction. But we still have not introduced peanuts to our older son who remains allergic to dairy and is now seven. Why would we do this? Why not give his digestive system a chance to fully heal itself before introducing this potentially dangerous food. The same goes for all tree nuts in our household.

Better safe than sorry. I was pleased to see Dr. Braly make this recommendation as well, *"We therefore generally recommend that parents refrain from giving their children peanut butter or other peanut or nut products until after they're two years old. If there is a family history of food allergies, parents should wait until the child is three. And many doctors recommend that their pregnant patients—*

especially those with food allergies—keep the lid on the peanut butter jar until after the baby is born and they've finished breast-feeding...at least until six months..." [25]

Roundtable Questions

1. Did you consider food allergies when you were pregnant?

2. If you did consider them, did you avoid the allergen foods or not?

3. In retrospect, would you change what you did or did not do and if so why?

4. Do you think taking probiotics when pregnant will actually improve the chances of not having an allergic child?

5. What other pregnancy concerns did you have that may or may not have impacted your child's allergies?

Toxic Load

Now that the new school year is well underway and the holidays are on the horizon, keeping our lives in balance is the challenge. There are many things that our boys want to do and many things that my husband and I want them and us to do, but the challenge is finding the priorities and the balance. When things get out of balance and we take on too much, the result is exhaustion, poor behavior, illness and toxic overload.

As any parent knows, balancing school, homework, baseball, piano, play dates and free time can be difficult when there are only twenty-four hours in a day. Allowing the daytime activities to sneak into bedtime and reduce nighttime sleeping hours never works—a short term gain in accomplishments leads to a long term loss in effectiveness from being exhausted.

Food allergies are an immune system disorder. I believe that when the immune system is stressed by exhaustion, emotional needs or illness the body then further succumbs to illness. I've found the old wives tales of keeping healthy to be quite effective. Specifically, *"don't get a chill," "get plenty of sleep," "eat right,"* and *"keeping a good attitude"* can impact the body's ability to handle the exposure to viruses the come through sneezes and coughing from schoolmates.

Our older son puts a lot of pressure on himself to help others and be a leader in school. But he pays the price in exhaustion after school. As we were waiting at the bus stop last week, he told me how tired he was, how his legs and back ached. His little chin trembled a bit as he told me and he looked a bit pale. My heart ached as I wondered what to do. Is he getting sick? Should I keep him home today? I'd have to call work and not go in as well. Was there a compromise? That's the constant struggle I feel when trying to do the right thing for my children. We decided he would go to school, but I picked him up a little early so he could avoid the bus ride home and spend an extra hour on the sofa eating and relaxing. I think it helped—he was tired at the end of the day, but felt better the next day.

I find that the medical studies and often many physicians dispute these sort of esoteric factors that a mother or father might take into consideration when deciding how to best take care of her child. I often read or hear, *"There is no medical basis,"* or *"There is no proof,"* with the undertone of *"you are being silly, woman."* But I believe and see evidence of these intangible factors as being significant. A person's body isn't just a composite of parts, but a whole. Understanding that one system impacts another that impacts yet another is important when it comes to health.

That's where the toxic load evolves: The more 'toxins' we put upon our bodies or our children's bodies, the harder the immune system must work to overcome them. This stress can negatively impact the body's ability to handle allergic reactions as well. It can reportedly make the reactions up to 200% worse at times of high stress according to some studies.

So I believe that striving to keep our lives in balance is of utmost importance for health at many different levels—emotional and physical as it pertains to illness and allergies, both of which rely on a strong immune system that itself can reach a more healthy level of balance by not overreacting to allergens and by being strong enough to fight off the true enemies in the world of viruses and unhealthy bacteria. Finding balance in a nebulous world of issues and outcomes is a true challenge for parents.

Roundtable Questions

1. What percentage of the time do you feel overwhelmed with your life and all of its activities?

2. If you are to cut out an activity, what is the first thing to which you would be willing to say, "No"?

3. Is your child one that thrives on activity or does he/she like quieter days?

4. After a busy day, how does your child act and how do you act, especially compared to quiet days?

5. Can you see any link between stress levels, illnesses and allergies?

Eczema and the Skin

When my first son was born he had cradle cap—patchy pieces on his scalp which I tried to oil and wash off painstakingly. He also developed a rash on his stomach, then on his arms and legs. I creamed this using a prescription cream from the doctor. Had I known better then I'd would have stopped eating and drinking dairy products—as he turned out to have a dairy allergy that has lasted for seven years thus far. I breastfed him and believe that the protein from dairy irritated his body. I often also wonder what other kind of discomfort it caused him. Did it give him cramps? Gas? Make him cry more? I finally figured out he had a dairy allergy and removed all dairy before he was a year old. His eczema was greatly reduced though his skin was still a bit dry, especially in the winter. Now, for the past year, since introducing fish oil into his diet, his dry skin isn't a problem at all. We occasionally use a little cream, but mostly just on his hands and only in the winter.

I've heard friends talking about the oozing red rash behind their child's elbow or knee. Or they talk of the variety of creams they've tried. One of the mothers interviewed in *Flourishing with Food Allergies* was so adamant about finding the *cause* of the eczema or rash on her infant that kept him and her up at night for weeks from the probable burning and itching feelings that she asked herself and her doctor over and over until she found the solution herself. She found her son was allergic to dairy and by removing it from her own diet she saw his eczema *"clear up by ninety percent."*

Sometimes the discovery can take place by accident. In Robyn O'Brien's book, *The Unhealthy Truth*, she discovered her son's eczema cleared up when they went on vacation and he didn't drink the many cups of milk that he normally consumed. Upon returning home and to his old habits, the eczema returned, as well as his cough and earaches. Eventually Robyn weaned him from milk, yogurt, cheese and other dairy products, which healed him.[26]

Over the years, I read a lot about itchy, red, bumpy rashes to try to understand why eczema and food allergies are created. I developed the following layperson's understanding: Eczema is caused by the inability of the infant's immature digestive system (or a child's or adult's digestive system) to breakdown certain proteins, such as the dairy proteins, which can be hard to digest. These stubborn proteins travel through the digestive system and go into the blood stream undigested. The liver then tries to cleanse the blood stream of this undigested protein. This works for a while, but then the liver becomes overloaded and cannot clean the bloodstream sufficiently. As a result, the immune system comes to the rescue and builds antibodies to attack the foreign proteins. Once the immune system creates antibodies, the allergic reaction is in place. The immune system's antibodies tell the body to attack that foreign substance as if it were a virus or disease, which can cause the body to go into overdrive, possibly resulting in anaphylactic shock, or less severe yet equally devastating delayed allergic responses that can contribute to asthma, ADHD or autism. In the meantime, this foreign substance still needs to be excreted from the infant's body, so the skin is used for excretion rather than the digestive system. Thus the skin becomes the cleanser of the body and shows a rash as the foreign substance comes out.[27]

I am sure that other things can irritate the skin. Environmental factors such as pets, dust mites, pollen can all contribute and make eczema worse, not to mention that there are other unrelated rashes caused by things like poison ivy. But I think people often overlook the fact that much of eczema can be caused by the food allergies to dairy, eggs, wheat, soy, peanuts, tree nuts, fish and shellfish. No matter how old you are or your child are—it can be a worthwhile experience to try to eliminate these foods for a week and see what happens. If nothing seems to change, try eliminating a different food for the next week. You may be pleasantly surprised at what problems you can solve without any medication or cost.

Roundtable Questions

1. Do you or does your child have any skin or rash issues?

2. Do you attempt to heal the cause or the symptom of these skin problems?

3. Do you think that the creams applied to skin can be absorbed into the skin and travel in the body?

4. Since your skin is the third major elimination organ in your body (after bowel/bladder) how could you improve the level of toxins that come out of your or your child's skin?

5. Would you consider eliminating a food for several weeks to watch the eczema to skin relationship?

Antibiotics

Our first son has taken a lot of antibiotics. At the age of six months he came down with strep, bronchitis and a sinus infection. At age two, he came down with pneumonia. Afterward up to age five he continued with about six rounds of antibiotics a year, give or take, for various sinus, ear and bronchial infections. We didn't know what else to do besides give him the antibiotics—he would develop such terrible coughs and we were so worried much of the time. It caused a great deal of stress, angst and concern for my husband and me.

Recently, Dr. David Schultz, a licensed clinical psychologist and lecturer at Yale University's School of Medicine, provided me with an interesting piece of literature that in part addresses the hygiene hypothesis as it relates to antibiotics. The excerpt taken from the book, *The Vaccination Dilemma* by Christine Murphy provides various perspectives on childhood vaccinations. In that book, Dr. Philip Incao states, *"Research has revealed a list of factors...that correlate with decreased risk of asthma and allergies, including the avoidance of vaccinations and antibiotics [such as] having little or no antibiotics especially before the age of two."* He continues, *"If the hygiene hypothesis proves to be correct, it will have a revolutionary impact on the medical practice...There is an ecology of human illness. If we attempt to eliminate a single element of an ecological system, we disturb the balance of the whole in ways that can lead to unforeseen consequences. To these unforeseen consequences belong the dramatic increases in asthma, allergies, diabetes, autism and learning dysfunctions occurring in children today."*[28]

Up to this point, it appeared to me that the hygiene hypothesis focused mainly on the child's external environment. But the internal world of bacteria within the child's body makes more sense to me. When that world is disturbed, repeatedly, with little or no effort to reconstitute or repopulate the beneficial bacteria, through the use of probiotics, like acidophilus in yogurt or non-dairy supplements, then that environment can become unbalanced and new problems can emerge.

I recall a passage from Dr. Kenneth Bock's book, *Healing the New Childhood Epidemics*, which states, *"There are two different kinds of helper T-cells: Th-1 and Th-2. The Th-1 cells...attack pathogens directly, or send messages to encourage other immune cells to attack. The Th-2 cells also attack pathogens but in a different way...by encouraging other immune cells to produce antibodies...then attack foreign substances, including bacteria, viruses and also allergens...Because these Th-1 and Th-2 cells work together, it's important that they stay in balance. But this doesn't always happen...there is a skewing of this balance, with an increase of Th-2 antibody production and a decrease of the activity of the Th-1 cells...The skewing of immunity to the Th-2 dominance makes it harder for people to fight off the viral, bacterial and fungal infections that lie within their cells. It makes them prone to many common illnesses. The excess activity of the Th-2 cells also triggers and overactive immune response with can result in allergy and autoimmunity...Overactive Th-2 immunity results in too many attacks on the substances that don't need to be attacked, including pollen and common foods such as milk and wheat. The final result is allergy. Allergy triggers inflammation as the body fights to free itself from presumed invaders. When the inflammation strikes the airways, asthma can occur."[29]*

In other words, the T-cells can become out of balance where one kind is weak and the other is overactive. The weak one can't fight off illness, like it should, while the overactive one overreacts causing unnecessary inflammation and allergic reactions. This described our son so well: He would get sick, we'd give him antibiotics which would enable the T-cell to remain weak rather than rising-to-the-challenge to fight off the illness. By continually giving him the antibiotics his T-cells would remain out of balance and the T-cell responsible for inflammation/allergies would never be reigned-in, put-in-check or calmed down.

Another problem with antibiotics is that leaky-gut can occur when the intestine walls become holey from an overgrowth of bad yeast or candida which can be caused by antibiotics killing off all bacteria (good and bad). When this happens, food particles that normally would be contained in the intestine leak out into the blood stream. The body is called upon to fight or deal with these food proteins. Immune systems come to the rescue but can cause immediate-IgE-food-allergies. Or in other bodies delayed-IgG-food-allergies are created leading to symptoms of the disorders of autism, ADHD or asthma.

Interestingly, our son was started on antibiotics just about the time I tried (unsuccessfully) to introduce cow's milk formula, to which he developed an allergy. The downward spiral in health continued for the next five years where he often fell into various infections after a regular cold. His ability to fight illness became worse and worse. I remember being in the toy store on the cold winter day of his fifth birthday asking him to pick out a favorite toy. We had just returned from the doctor for the painful-to-listen-to non-stop cough he had developed. All he could choke out was, "*Get the castle book*" and we quickly went home. I felt so terrible for him.

Mostly because of what I learned from researching *Flourishing with Food Allergies* and interviewing the parents and doctors, we were finally able to pull out of this cycle. I summoned up the courage to call a recommended naturopath doctor, a kind of medicine with which I had no personal experience and felt somewhat skeptical. This new doctor gave our son supplements to detoxify his body from mucus and reduce respiratory inflammation as well as improve the strength of his immune system. We started this in March. During April his congestion drained like never before. I literally ran around the park one spring day with a box of tissues chasing after him to blow his nose every few minutes—and I was quite happy about it. By May his mucus cleared, a chronic cough finally completely subsided and his breathing at night was tremendously quiet! Previously, I used to be able to 'check on him' at the bottom of the stairs—I could hear him breathing and snorkeling from that far away. It was so stressful to hear this every night for my husband and me. But then, in May, I remember the night when I walked into his doorway and couldn't hear him. I became worried and took steps closer to his bed and heard him breathing so peacefully. It is still a joy to listen to him at night and remains our favorite recurring topic of conversation between my husband and me.

This new naturopath doctor also explained to me that in addition to clearing mucus and decreasing inflammation using natural supplements and tonics he would work to strengthen our son's immune system. Having read the passage above from Dr. Bock's book about T-cells this made sense to me, i.e. reduce inflammation while improving immune response. It is my hope that by rebalancing his immune system his ability to fight illness will be corrected and his overreaction to the allergy-foods will eventually diminish and go away. After five months on the treatment we had a skin prick test. His allergies to dairy and egg remained, but were much less than the previous year. His dairy went from the size of a quarter to a dime. The egg went from the size of a dime to an eraser top. Another benefit that is intangible but immense is that his mood improved, within a few weeks. I don't need to tell mothers how much easier life is when your child comes up for the bath on the first call rather than turning it into another 'issue.'

Over the past eight months under the supervision of both of my son's doctors (naturopathic and allopathic) he has been on antibiotics only once for strep throat. He has had many colds/viruses and even a mild ear ache and few fevers, but has recovered from them on his own. At first, my husband and I were fearful, then amazed, as we watched him conquer these invisible wars. It is our hope that his body rebalances. If his T-cells balance out perhaps he will outgrow his allergy faster. We will use antibiotics when an infection is serious, but will try quite hard to avoid them up to that point.

In closing, my thoughts about antibiotics are as follows. I believe antibiotics are important in the effort to help the body recover from serious illness. But the over-use of antibiotics can deplete the child's (or anyone's) natural and good bacteria supply in their gut and also disrupt the body's T-cell balance causing problems in naturally fighting illness. While the bacterial supply can be remedied by supplementing with probiotics, there is a longer term negative effect by way of leaky gut which probably causes the more permanent food allergies. Further, how do you strengthen the T-cell that has become weak due to overuse of antibiotics? Letting it work it out by fighting the illness itself seems to be the only way. It is like tough love—letting your loved one struggle because in the end that's the best thing for them.

We are now quite careful to use antibiotics only when it is necessary such as for a high fever, strep throat, pneumonia, or other serious life-threatening and/or permanently damaging illness.

Roundtable Questions

1. Should children be given antibiotics at the first sign of a problem or should they try to tough it out?

2. Do you believe antibiotics are over-prescribed—how often has your child received them?

3. Do you think that antibiotics can lead to intestinal issues, like leaky gut, which then give way to food allergies?

4. Do you think there could be a link between leaky gut syndrome and autism, ADHD or asthma?

5. Where do you draw the line for when to take antibiotics or not, or do you rely completely on your doctor?

Leaky Gut

What is leaky gut or leaky gut syndrome? According to Dr. Weil's book, *Leaky Gut Syndrome*, *"[Leaky gut] is the result of damage to the intestinal lining, making it less able to protect the internal environment as well as to filter needed nutrients and other biological substances. As a consequence, some bacteria and their toxins, incompletely digested proteins and fats, and waste not normally absorbed may 'leak' out of the intestines into the blood stream. This triggers an autoimmune reaction, which can lead to gastrointestinal problems such as abdominal bloating, excessive gas and cramps, fatigue, food sensitivities, joint pain, skin rashes, and autoimmunity...Leaky gut syndrome may trigger or worsen such disorders as Crohn's disease, celiac disease, rheumatoid arthritis and asthma."*[30]

Research has caused me to believe that leaky gut can lead to food allergies (and contribute to autism). We know food allergies are an immune system response to food proteins. The most common food proteins that cause food allergies are dairy, egg, soy, wheat, egg, tree nuts, peanuts, fish and shell fish. It is my understanding that when a child is exposed to one (or more) of these allergens, a food allergy can be triggered especially if that child had leaky gut syndrome. While most doctors do not test for leaky gut syndrome and because it is invisible to the eye, a parent must rely on symptoms. As Dr. Weil states, rashes are a symptom and you can see a rash on your child. Other symptoms may be hard to identify because children cannot effectively communicate how they feel. An infant can't tell you that he or she has gas, cramps, pain or trouble breathing. But a skin rash is obvious and can be the offending protein making its way out of the body through the skin. My first son had cradle cap and skin rashes on his arms, legs and occasionally his back and face.

Another symptom can be thrush or candida overgrowth—more commonly known as yeast. While a 'yeast infection' is something women usually think about with respect to reproductive health, it can equally affect the digestive track. The National Candida Center explains, *"Candida overgrowth (candida albicans) can lead to candida yeast infection and leaky gut syndrome which is medically referred to as intestinal permeability. Leaky gut is a major gastrointestinal disorder that occurs when openings develop in the gut wall. These tiny holes can be created when candida overgrowth moves to a more serious stage of candida yeast infection and the candida yeast grows roots or hypha (plural hyphae) which is a long, branching filamentous cell of a fungus. This fungal growth is a more advanced stage of development in the candida albicans yeast infection. The hyphae spreads the bowel wall cells apart so that acidic, harmful microorganisms and macromolecules are then able to pass through (leak) these openings and enter the circulatory system—why it is called 'leaky gut.' The body is alerted to the invader and creates antibodies for protection, activates the immune system, and thus is born a food allergy. Food allergies are directly linked to leaky gut and candida yeast infection overgrowth.*"[31]

For years, my first son had a lot of white stuff on his tongue. We'd try to brush it off and use mouthwash, but it would reappear. Our current doctor identified it as candida. After one and one-half years on a probiotic regimen prescribed by our doctor and careful rinsing of toothbrushes with a hydrogen peroxide-based mouthwash, my son's tongue is finally a beautiful pink. It is my hope that if his intestines are now healed from a candida overgrowth then perhaps his body will outgrow his dairy and egg allergy. He just turned eight years old this past January and while he has made progress in the severity of his reactions over the past seven years, the allergy still exists (mild to moderate according to the skin prick test results). While I have no proof as to the cause of the candida problem, it is my opinion that too many antibiotics during infancy and toddler years without replenishment of probiotics, set him up for food allergies. In fact, I remember that when he was six months old, he had his first round of antibiotics. Around that time, I tried to wean him from breast milk to cow's milk-based formula—thus producing our first allergic reaction.

If I had to do it over again, and know what I know now, I'd find a doctor who used antibiotics sparingly and who would have recommended a probiotics supplement for my child, especially after the use of antibiotics. Ironically, the use of probiotics can also help fight off illness and boost the immune system as well—so the need for antibiotics is reduced.

Roundtable Questions

1. Do you think that doctors should offer to test for leaky gut syndrome?

2. How could leaky gut be tested? Blood tests? Bowel tests?

3. Do you think intestinal problems can lead to allergies?

4. Do you think intestinal problems can lead to other problems such as arthritis, asthma, autism, ADHD?

5. Would you supplement with probiotics to avoid leaky gut or candida/yeast infections in the digestive tract?

Autism, ADHD and Asthma

How can food allergies affect children who have the disorders of autism, ADHD and asthma?

There are (at least) two types of antibodies that can be created by a child's body: IgE and IgG. The IgE antibody normally produces an *immediate*-food-allergy reaction. The IgG antibody normally produces a *delayed*-food-allergy reaction (think of the 'G' for gradual or delayed).

Immediate-food-allergy reactions can produce hives and anaphylaxis (swelling of the lips, tongue and throat along with trouble breathing). Reactions normally occur within a few minutes of eating the offending food, but can take up to 24-hours to occur.

Delayed-food-allergy reactions normally take *at least a few hours or days* to occur. The symptoms of this type of reaction can be more difficult to spot. Reportedly, delayed-food-allergy reactions can be responsible for the behavioral disorders of autism and ADHD as well as reactions of asthma.

Consider Dr. Kenneth Bock's thoughts in his book, *Healing the New Childhood Epidemics* where he states, *"A very significant advantage of blood testing, as opposed to skin testing, is that it reveals the presence of IgG reactions. IgG reactions typically don't show up during skin testing, because they often don't begin to occur until a few hours, or even a few days, after contact with the food. In contrast, IgE reactions generally occur almost immediately, enabling doctors to spot them during the short duration of the skin testing procedure. IgG reactions are very common, and very troublesome. They are extremely common among kids with 4-A disorders: Autism, ADHD, Asthma and Allergies. They tend to create less severe symptoms than IgE reactions, but their symptoms still can be extremely destructive, particularly when IgG reactions to several foods occur at once, causing combined, cumulative damage, or when they combine with IgE reactions."*[32]

While hives and eczema can be symptoms of immediate-reaction food allergy, it is behavioral issues that are a symptom of delayed-reaction food allergy. As Dr. Josef Burton explains in *Flourishing with Food Allergies*, *"Reactions can be both visible and invisible. We can see rashes and hives, but there are reactions that are not as easy to identify such as grumpiness and irritability. If a child's tongue or lips can swell, why can't his brain swell too? Offending foods probably make our internal organs swell at times that can make it difficult or nearly impossible for a child to do the things we expect, such as sit and study or act the way we expect him to act."* [33]

When an undigested protein particle gets through the intestine walls it goes into the blood stream and the immune system is called upon to 'handle it.' Depending upon the child, his or her body breaks down this protein particle the best it can. But during this breakdown process there can be side effects from the chemicals produced by the child's own body. For instance, Dr. Scot Lewey writes on autism, *"Many parents report a casein-free (dairy protein) and gluten-free diet increases eye contact, attention, and mood while decreasing aggressive or oppositional behavior, tantrums, and poor attention. Theories for improvement of casein-free diet include improved brain function due to removal of cow's milk protein by-products that have opiate-like effects. Casomorphin is protein fragment or peptide sequence derived from casein that is considered to have an opiate like effect. There are several casomorphins produced by digestion of casein from cow's milk. People who stop eating wheat and dairy containing foods commonly report withdrawal symptoms."* [34]

People who crave certain foods are actually feeding a negative circle of addiction to something that is harmful for their particular bodies. Specifically, *"[A]ddictive cravings and withdrawal symptoms are said to exist in many food allergy patients when they stop eating the offending foods. It has been suggested that this may be because some protein fragments formed when food is broken down are similar to endorphins, which the body produces naturally to counteract pain and produce euphoria. Then the allergy sufferer's body becomes adapted to that level of endorphin activity and so craves the allergen in order to maintain the endorphin levels."* [35]

Common delayed-reaction allergy foods include:

- **ADHD/ADD**: Dairy, wheat, oranges, eggs, chocolate, artificial colorings, artificial flavorings, food preservatives and natural chemicals found in apricots, berries and tomatoes.

- **Autism**: Dairy, wheat, gluten, caffeine, chocolate, artificial colorings, artificial flavorings, soy and corn.

- **Asthma**: Dairy, wheat, egg, yeast, preservatives, colorings and coffee.

The above list is taken from Dr. Kenneth Bock's book.[36] He details nutritional supplements to boost the immune system and cleanse the body from heavy metals that can lodge in brain tissues and disrupt normal functioning. Supplementing properly can result in improving and often eliminating the symptoms and behavior associated with ADHD and autism, which Dr. Bock places on the same spectrum. Additional research, studies, interviews and examples of improving symptoms of asthma, ADHD and autism can be found in *Flourishing with Food Allergies*, in chapters dedicated to those topics. To test your child for delayed-reactions, you must do a blood test. (The skin prick test can only find immediate allergic reactions.) Blood tests can locate both the IgG (delayed) and IgE (immediate) antibodies. You'll need to locate an allergist who understands this and can order and evaluate the results, hopefully with insurance coverage.

Roundtable Questions

1. What is the difference between an immediate IgE allergy and a delayed IgG allergy?

2. Is this difference identifiable through a skin prick test or only a blood test?

3. Do you think that IgG allergies can contribute to autism, ADHD or asthma?

4. If IgG allergies cause swelling or other internal reactions how can you determine whether they are impacting you or your child?

5. Would you be willing to avoid a food for several weeks to detoxify the body and see if there is a difference in behavior or other symptoms?

Seasonal Allergies

While it is normally a bit of a challenge to keep up with the food allergy related issues of children—preparing for birthday parties, making lunches daily and carefully scanning all ingredients—the springtime with seasonal allergies has increased our stress load and therefore had an emotional impact on us.

Every spring our older son's eyes get a little itchy and red and he may become congested, but I now realize that the past has been mild to moderate compared to this year. Five weeks ago, we kicked off the allergy season with a Monday of red, swollen, itchy eyes. Since then he has avoided going outside despite the beautiful spring weather. He has been diligent about showering before bed to wash off pollen, especially when he has been outside for baseball practice. Despite our carefulness, it has been difficult, to say the least.

His eyes remain itchy and swollen. We give him eye drops, but I worry about putting so many drops in those beautiful blue eyes. I also wonder about the side effects of eye drops—what is dripping into his sinus cavity? Could it be making him even stuffier? Could all of the eye rubbing give him an infection? Are his nails short enough? Are his hands clean?

Then there is the congestion: His nose is stuffy beyond belief. We give him antihistamine but depending upon the type, the medicine either makes him tired or jumpy. Plus, once the antihistamine wears wear off—there are more side effects. Specifically, his sleep is disrupted or his congestion increases even more than it may have otherwise—the dependency factor.

But by far, the scariest seasonal allergy symptom is the trouble breathing. For the first time this year the school nurse called me—I was one hour from the school—she advised me that my son was having trouble breathing. He was wheezing. As every parent can imagine, my stress level sky rocketed as I tried not to race down the highway to the school. By the time I arrived, he seemed better, much better. So we went home and tried to relax.

But by bed time he started coughing and by ten o'clock he was coughing violently while sleeping—to the point of almost vomiting. Terribly worried, I called his pediatrician and he told us to give our son some medication through the nebulizer as well as some oral medication to stop the wheezing and coughing. I must admit that although we use medications sparingly instead trying to allow his body to heal itself through more natural vitamins like fish oil and probiotics, these medications worked beautifully. Within ten minutes he was breathing deeply and there was no more coughing.

So these three springtime symptoms of seasonal allergies over the past five weeks have impacted us emotionally. Our son is frustrated—tired of it all. He has even starting to complain—normally he stoically handles food allergies—eating non-dairy and non-egg foods at lunch and parties. Now he has begun to ask, *"Why doesn't my brother have pollen allergies?"* The undertone of, *"This isn't fair!"* is coming across stronger and stronger. His personality has also changed a bit by giving into less patience and more frustration with everyday things.
 Normally he can be so loving and quite charming but I can see how frustrated he is—at the end of his rope. The symptoms are relentless.

I have been worrying a lot—getting up several times some nights to check on his breathing. I feel so bad for him—wishing that I could adopt his stuffy nose and let him relax and breathe freely. I pray for rain—watching the weather report hoping for a cleansing downpour. I tell him that many, many people have to deal with seasonal allergies, but I still feel terrible for him. I tell him how things could be even harder—that we should appreciate his otherwise good health and strong abilities. I list off those things he does so well...baseball, piano, math, friendships, helping others...I think it makes him feel better at the moment. Advising him to, *"Hang in there,"* and *"Never give up hope,"* helps him believe that things will get better—just around the corner. They will.

He is a trooper. I am proud because I know how hard he tries to participate in all he can. I take solace in knowing that he will do well in life because he can work through the toughest times. He can play baseball with a head full of stuffiness—and hit the ball *hard* time after time on the first swing. He can do his homework day after day while tired and crabby—and still get it all correct. He can perk up and enjoy his weekly piano lesson. He can put a big, marvelous smile on his face for others—even in spite of his struggles and allergies. Keeping one's proverbial chin up is a lifelong skill that will help him. Perhaps things will really get better today. It finally rained last night.

Roundtable Questions

1. Do you or does someone you love get seasonal allergies?

2. Do doctors or people dismiss the impact of season allergies by saying, *"it is just allergies"* and how does this make you feel?

3. How do the allergies impact your state of mind when you are working or dealing with every day things?

4. Is there anything 'nice' that you can do for yourself or child during this time, besides medication, to make yourself happier (i.e. a treat of a massage for yourself or a special gift for your child.)

5. Would you considering taking allergy drops or having treatments to try to improve the situation?

Gluten and Celiac Disease

In mid-March, I begin to think about spring allergies. Last year my oldest son, now nine, suffered a lot. He wheezed—which never happened before. His eyes were itchy, red and swollen—something with which we are accustom. There was also congestion, of course. But by far, the most worrisome was the wheezing, which left me standing by his bedside as he slept while coughing and wheezing while I spoke with his pediatrician over the telephone at ten o'clock in the evening. Under the advice of the pediatrician, I gave him some breathing treatments that we had and it helped a great deal.

This year have a new reason for being hopeful. Under the guidance of a naturopathic physician, we learned through a delayed ('IgG') allergy test, that my sons are both sensitive or have a delayed allergy to gluten (wheat and rye). He advised us to remove gluten from our diets. Three weeks ago today, I gave away our wheat pasta, replacing it with rice pasta. After much searching, my husband found a gluten-free bread that did not contain egg or dairy—not an easy task. (I tried making the bread in my bread maker but it was about as hard as a softball.)

I noticed that after one week of giving up gluten, I felt awful. I was tired, crabby and foggy. My younger son reported that he had a headache—something unusual for a seven year old. My older son succumbed to a terrible cold after two weeks with much congestion. Of course it is difficult to determine if the backlash from the gluten-free diet contributed to a temporary increase in inflammation in his sinuses.

Now three weeks later, we are okay (I think). Plus we are hopeful—the naturopath doctor said that people who have a delayed allergy to gluten suffer from increased inflammation and worsened seasonal allergies. He said that a patient of his would end up in the hospital each spring for breathing trouble, until the year he removed gluten from his diet. That year, he was okay—the inflammation did not exist.

So as we approach April and May, I will wait and watch my son. There are so many factors such as the amount of pollen in the air that it will be hard to draw a final conclusion. But I am hopeful that there will be an improvement in his seasonal allergies through the preventative measure of removing gluten from his diet.

Roundtable Questions

1. While most doctors/insurance companies don't support the IgG delayed allergy test, do you believe it is valid?

2. Would you be willing to remove gluten from your diet for three solid weeks to see if there is a change in how you or your child feels?

3. Do you find that you or your child just "*loves*" bread and pasta?

4. Do you think it would be too hard and subjective to remove gluten and to see any changes?

5. Would you prefer to have a celiac blood test—rather than removing the gluten?

Parasites Causing Food Allergies

Yes, parasites. Just the word makes most of us shiver. Some people will even refuse to discuss or think about them. While we are more comfortable with parasites existing in animals, such as tapeworms dogs and cats, the fact is that most people probably have parasites too—even in the United States, Europe and other developed areas of the world. Doctors such as the well-known TV personality Dr. Oz; Dr. Ross Anderson, a parasitic infection specialist and author; Dr. Peter Wina, Chief of Patho-Biology in the Walter Reed Army Institute of Research; and Dr. Frank Nova, Chief of the Laboratory for Parasitic Diseases of the National Institute of Health have all been quoted making statements that generally indicate as many as 85% to 95% of adults probably have parasites.

According to the USDA, *"Young children, pregnant women, older adults, and persons with weakened immune systems, are highly susceptible to parasites for several reasons. First, because the immune systems are weaker than most adults the parasite isn't eliminated easily. Second, children are often on the ground and putting things into their mouths that may not be clean, specifically things that may have come into contact with animal or human feces. Third, children may accidentally swallow pool or lake water that is contaminated since many parasites can live for several days in chlorinated water. Fourth, young children in daycare can easily contract parasites from other children through shared diaper changing facilities. Fifth, eating raw, unwashed fruits and vegetables or eating undercooked meats can deliver parasites directly into human bodies."*[37]

But how can parasites play a part in allergies, especially food allergies? According to Dr. Leo Galland, *"One of the most common effects of intestinal parasites is food allergy. I looked at the effects of parasitic infection among patients in my medical practice. For people with multiple food allergies who were found to have intestinal parasites, treatment of the parasitic infection produced a dramatic reduction in food allergy in about half the cases. It's my belief that anyone with food intolerance or allergy should be tested for intestinal parasites...Parasites may cause allergic or autoimmune disorders in two ways. First, the inflammation caused by an intestinal infection can cause an increase in the permeability of the small intestine, a phenomenon known colloquially as 'leaky gut'...Second, over two-thirds of your body's immune system is located in the wall of the small intestine. The immune cells (called lymphocytes) leave the intestine and travel all over your body. When activated by a parasitic infection, they can carry the inflammatory message to your joints, your skin, your eyes, and your lungs."* [38]

In summary, parasites can weaken the immune system and cause overreactions to otherwise harmless substances such as food allergens of soy, wheat, egg, dairy, peanuts, tree nuts, fish and shell fish. If a parent thinks that parasites might be a contributing factor to their child's food allergies, then that parent could locate a doctor who understands and can treat a child for parasites. It may take several phone calls or visits to find a doctor that is educated in this area by being able to explain the appropriate tests and medications to rid the child's body of parasites.

Roundtable Questions

1. Can you think of any time that you or your child may have come into contact with parasites (e.g. animal feces, sandboxes, lake swimming, undercooked food)?

2. Do you have a pet that has been treated for parasites?

3. Would you consider going to the doctor for a parasite test?

4. Would you consider taking a remedy sold at stores?

5. Do you think there is any relationship between food allergies and parasites?

Carrots can Kill Parasites

"Where's my carrot juice?!" my eight year-old exclaimed as he marched in the kitchen at seven o'clock this morning on the fifth day of summer. Miracles do happen. We are on a carrot-juice-kick for the summer—freshly made each morning, one pound of washed, organic carrots yields about three to four ounces each for the three of us. The first day was a struggle—"*Eawww! Gross!*" My older son had a bad (mostly psychological) reaction—felt sick to his stomach—we discovered from gulping it down he had too much air in his stomach. The complaining lasted for about 15 minutes. The second day was (a little) easier—complaining for only about five minutes. The third was somewhat of a surrender...

This summer I want the kids to get sunshine, exercise, rest and a lot of good, natural nutrients. I've read that carrot juice has everything from beta-carotene, vitamin A, PP, B1, B2, E, potassium, calcium, sodium, magnesium, iron and phosphorus.[39] It is even supposed to help people with weak immune systems. Bingo! Allergies are a symptom of a weak immune system. Anything I can do to help improve that for my children is on top of my list.

According to the United Kingdom's World Carrot Museum web site, "*Carrots help to keep your immune system strong Vitamin A is essential for the proper functioning of the immune system. This nutrient keeps the skin and cells that line the airways, digestive tract and urinary tract healthy, so they act as barriers and form the body's first line of defense against infection.*"[40]

I also read that it is important not to drink too much of the carrot juice as it can overload, rather than cleanse, the liver. The correct amount of carrot juice can cleanse the liver—something so important for our kids with food and environmental allergies. According to the Idaho Observer, "*We have found that nearly all diseases can be 'cured' by improving the functioning of the liver, our body's chemical factory and organ of detoxification.*"[41] So if an adult can have eight ounces a day, I am giving my sons about three to four ounces a day. This seems to be the right amount in terms of how much they are willing to drink anyway.

Carrot juice also reportedly will kill off certain parasites, like pinworms—something little kids can pick up from other kids in day care, especially when they put things in their mouths. According to

India's Hpathy.com, *"Many allergies in humans are caused by worm infections. Tissue becomes inflamed and reactions to foods are the result when eosinophils (white blood cells) are increased due to them. Extreme skin rashes with blisters and food allergies or sensitivities may result."*[42]

Roundtable Questions

1. Would you be willing to drink fresh carrot juice to remove some parasites?

2. How long would you stick with a new plan to improve health for you or your child?

3. Should you confirm with a doctor before you begin a regimen?

4. Do you think that rashes and other strange symptoms could be caused by parasites?

5. Are you willing to think about this or does it just make your skin crawl?

Government Subsidies

While I know dairy isn't good for *my* children due to their allergy to it, I speculated it wasn't great for those of us who are not allergic to it either—isn't it meant for calves? After my second grade son came home from school last week asking about his 'food pyramid' lesson with respect to the importance of dairy, we laughed as its silliness and turned it into a game of, *"Why do people eat cow's milk? We don't eat horse's milk, or kangaroo's milk, or giraffe's milk..."* It was fun.

After our conversation, I recalled that the USDA was originally involved in the creation of the food pyramid. It appears the food pyramid was created in the 1990s—although I remember it earlier than that. Apparently food charts have been created back to the 1940s—in fact the, "Guide to Good Eating" shows that 1/7th of our intake should be butter or margarine—which just seems preposterous. But then again, smoking was widely popular then.

Now, decades later, the USDA is *still* involved in promoting dairy, even though they fully admit it causes health problems such as obesity. This weekend *The New York Times* came out with an article titled, *While Warning About Fat, U.S. Pushes Cheese Sales*[43] which explains the government's findings that dairy consumption causes obesity due to the high saturated fat content. But the hypocrisy is in the fact that another branch of the government is spending *millions* promoting supposed health benefits of dairy to unsuspecting Americans and even those overseas.

Specifically, there is a branch in the government that collects money from farmers and also uses tax payers' money to promote dairy. This Dairy Management Agency spends roughly $140 million each year managing dairy. For instance, they recently entered into a contract with Domino's Pizza to promote cheese and spent $12 million in doing so. Even overseas isn't safe from the promotion—$5.3 million was spent on that marketplace.

Even worse, the promotion and advertising is working. *"These efforts [the department reported] helped generate a cheese sales growth of nearly 30 million pounds."* Dairy consumption is way up, *"Americans now eat an average of 33 pounds of cheese a year, nearly triple the 1970 rate."*

Are those marketing jingles (Got Milk?) and claims (weight loss and improved health) true? *"Having dismissed the weight-loss claim in*

2005, the federal nutrition advisory committee this summer again found the underlying science 'not convincing.' The campaign lasted until 2007, when the Federal Trade Commission acted on a two-year-old petition by the Physicians Committee for Responsible Medicine, an advocacy group that challenged the campaign's claims. 'If you want to look at why people are fat today, it's pretty hard to identify a contributor more significant than this meteoric rise in cheese consumption,' Dr. Neal D. Barnard, president of the physicians' group, said in an interview."

So if our health is negatively impacted by dairy consumption, we all pay for it through our health insurance premiums. It seems so odd that the government would promote something that has been found to cause disease and many trickle down health issues. Maybe it was someone's idea for creating jobs for our economy.

Roundtable Questions

1. Do you think dairy products are healthy, if so why?

2. If calcium is the primary reason then did you know that more absorbable calcium can be obtained in vegetables?

3. Would you or your family be willing to give up dairy or is that out of the question?

4. Do you think the government should promote dairy so strongly or let the free market reign?

5. Do you think everyone who pays tax should pay for the promotion of dairy?

Acknowledgements

I'd like to thank my two sons for inspiring me to try to help others. Thank you to my husband who is so supportive. Thank you to my family and friends who show their support by making dairy and egg-free meals and snacks for us.

Disclaimer

The author of this book is not a doctor or medical professional. Neither the author nor publisher assumes any liability or responsibility for damage or injury to persons or property arising from any use of any product, information, idea or guidance contained in the materials provided. This book does not specifically recommend or endorse any test, products or procedures that have been mentioned. The contents of this book are not intended to provide medical advice. Medical advice should be obtained from a qualified health professional. No treatment action should be undertaken without consultation with a physician. The information should not be considered complete, nor should it be relied on to suggest a course of treatment for a particular individual. Some information may be out of date due to the rapidly changing nature of the field of food allergies.

End Notes

[1] Wikipedia, "Round Table," http://en.wikipedia.org/wiki/Round_Table

[2] Allen, JoAnne, "Studies confirm treatment may help peanut allergy," Reuters Health, 3/2010, http://in.mobile.reuters.com/article/health/idINTRE62056B20100301

[3] Institute for Agriculture and Trade Policy, "Much High Fructose Corn Syrup Contaminated With Mercury, New Study Finds," 1/2009, http://www.iatp.org/documents/much-high-fructose-corn-syrup-contaminated-with-mercury-new-study-finds

[4] Regush, Nicholas, "The Verge of Vaccine Mania," 2010, http://www.shirleys-wellness-cafe.com/vaccines.htm

[5] Emed Expert, "16 Interesting Facts About Antibiotics," 2010, http://www.emedexpert.com/tips/antibiotics-facts.shtml#ref3

[6] Autism Education Summit, "CDC Scientist Admits Cover-up of MMR/autism Causation Demand a Full Investigation by Congress," 9/5/2014, http://www.ageofautism.com/2014/09/cdc-scientist-admits-cover-up-of-mmrautism-causation-demand-a-full-investigation-by-congress.html

[7] Wikipedia, "Chelation therapy," http://en.wikipedia.org/wiki/Chelation_therapy

[8] "The Poor Man's Chelation Therapy," http://home.earthlink.net/~jedcline/cilantro.html

[9] Allergy & Asthma Network, "When Will I Outgrow Food Allergies?" 2/2009, http://www.aanma.org/2009/02/when-will-i-outgrow-food-allergies/

[10] About Health, "My Child is Allergic to Milk. When Might He Outgrow His Food Allergy?" 6/2014, http://allergies.about.com/od/fa1/f/outgrowmilk.htm

[11] FARE, "Who is Likely to Outgrow a Food Allergy?" 2013, http://blog.foodallergy.org/2013/09/13/who-is-likely-to-outgrow-a-food-allergy/

[12] American College of Allergy, Asthma & Immunology, "Tree Nut Allergy," http://www.acaai.org/allergist/allergies/Types/food-allergies/types/Pages/tree-nut-allergy.aspx

[13] Medical News Today, "9% of Children May Outgrow Their Tree Nut Allergies," 2005, http://www.medicalnewstoday.com/releases/33312.php

[14] The Wall Street Journal, "Is Your Kids Truly Allergic? Tests Add to Food Confusion," 2010, http://online.wsj.com/news/articles/SB10001424052748703808904575025011

3194645130?mg=reno64-
wsj&url=http%3A%2F%2Fonline.wsj.com%2Farticle%2FSB1000142405274870
380890457502501319464513O.html

[15] PubMed Health, "Omalizumab (Injection)," 8/2014,
http://www.ncbi.nlm.nih.gov/pubmedhealth/PMHT0011491/?report=details

[16] Drugs.com, "Omalizumab Side Effects,"
http://www.drugs.com/sfx/omalizumab-side-effects.html

[17] The Free Dictionary, "Caveat Emptor," http://legal-
dictionary.thefreedictionary.com/Buyer+beware

[18] Stanford Medicine News Center, "New treatment may desensitize kids with
milk allergies, say researchers," 3/2011, http://med.stanford.edu/news/all-
news/2011/03/new-treatment-may-desensitize-kids-with-milk-allergies-say-
researchers.html,

[19] Allergyhope.org, "Desensitization Treatment for Life-Threatening Food
Allergies," 2011, http://allergyhope.org/allergyhope/

[20] American Academy of Allergy Asthma & Immunology, "Challenge to baked
milk," 1/2012 http://www.aaaai.org/ask-the-expert/challenge-to-baked-
milk.aspx

[21] Health for Life Clinic, Dr. Ann Lee, N.D., "What is Homeopathy?"
http://www.doctornaturalmedicine.com/what-is-homeopathy

[22] Healio Infection Diseases in Children, "Could oral immunotherapy be the
first treatment for food allergy?" 9/2010,
http://www.healio.com/pediatrics/allergy-asthma-
immunology/news/online/%7Bf062c014-ec1c-4a73-8557-
28d07860c250%7D/could-oral-immunotherapy-be-the-first-treatment-for-
food-allergy

[23] Nowak-Wegrzyn, M.D., Anna, Fiocchi, A., "Is Oracle Immunotherapy the
Cure for Food Allergies," Allergy and Clinical Immunology, PubMed.gov,
6/2010, http://www.ncbi.nlm.nih.gov/pubmed/20431369

[24] Braley, M.D., James, Holford, Patrick, "Hidden Food Allergies," Basic Health
Publications, Inc., Laguna Beach, CA, originally published by Piatkus Books,
Ltd., Great Britain, London, England 2005, page 89.

[25] Braley, M.D., James, Holford, Patrick, "Hidden Food Allergies," Basic Health
Publications, Inc., Laguna Beach, CA, originally published by Piatkus Books,
Ltd., Great Britain, London, England 2005, page 69.

[26] O'Brien, Robyn, "The Unhealthy Truth," Broadway Books, NY, 2009, p 147-
150.

[27] Anderson, A. "Flourishing with Food Allergies," Papoose Publishing LLC, CT, 2008, p. 35.

[28] Murphy, Christine, Editor, "The Vaccination Dilemma", Lantern Books, 2000.

[29] Bock, M.D., Kenneth, Stauth, Cameron, "Healing the New Childhood Epidemics: Autism, ADHD, Asthma and Allergies. The Groundbreaking Program for the 4-A Disorders," Ballantine Books, an imprint of Random House, New York, NY, 2008.

[30] Weil, M.D., Andrew, "What is Leaky Gut?" Weil Lifestyle, LLC., 2/12/2005, http://www.drweil.com/drw/u/QAA361058/what-is-leaky-gut.html

[31] National Candida Center ,"Candida Yeast Infection Leaky Gut, Irritable Bowel and Food Allergies," 2014, http://www.nationalcandidacenter.com/leaky-gut/

[32] Bock, M.D., Kenneth, Stauth, Cameron, "Healing the New Childhood Epidemics: Autism, ADHD, Asthma and Allergies. The Groundbreaking Program for the 4-A Disorders," Ballantine Books, an imprint of Random House, New York, NY, 2008.

[33] Anderson, A., "Flourishing with Food Allergies," July 2008, Papoose Publishing LLC.

[34] Lewey, Dr. Scot, "Autism linked to cow's milk protein when GI symptoms present: More thoughts on the brain gut connection," 1/3/2007, http://thefooddoc.blogspot.com/search?q=Casomorphin+is+protein+fragment

[35] Thurnell-Read, Jane, "Allergy Equals Addiction," 11/10/2007, http://www.shareware123.com/articles/part9/allergy_equals_addiction.htm

[36] Bock, M.D., Kenneth, Stauth, Cameron, "Healing the New Childhood Epidemics: Autism, ADHD, Asthma and Allergies. The Groundbreaking Program for the 4-A Disorders," Ballantine Books, an imprint of Random House, New York, NY, 2008.

[37] USDA's Foodborne Illness & Disease, "Parasites and Foodborne Illness," 5/24/2011 , http://www.fsis.usda.gov/wps/portal/fsis/topics/food-safety-education/get-answers/food-safety-fact-sheets/foodborne-illness-and-disease/parasites-and-foodborne-illness/

[38] Galland, M.D., Leo, "What's Living in Your Digestive System?" Huffington Post, 3/2/2011, http://www.huffingtonpost.com/leo-galland-md/stomach-parasites_b_828565.html

[39] Health by Nature.com, "Carrot Juice Benefits, Nutrition Facts & Side Effects," 4/2013, http://myhealthbynature.com/carrot-juice-benefits-side-effects/

[40] The Carrot Museum, "The Health Benefits of Carrots," 2014, http://www.carrotmuseum.co.uk/healthbenefits.html

[41] Cassel, Ingri, "Carrot juice: Key to rejuvenating the liver," 5/2007, http://www.proliberty.com/observer/20070506.htm

[42] Hpathy Ezine, "Parasites in Humans & their Symptoms – Tapeworm, roundworm, pinworms," 8/2009 http://hpathy.com/cause-symptoms-treatment/worms-intestinal-worms-in-humans/

[43] Moss, Micheal, The New York Times, "While Warning About Fat, U.S. Pushes Cheese Sales," 11/6/2010, http://www.nytimes.com/2010/11/07/us/07fat.html?_r=3&pagewanted=all

www.ingramcontent.com/pod-product-compliance
Lightning Source LLC
Chambersburg PA
CBHW050120280326
41933CB00010B/1182